Adhesive Technology for Restorative Dentistry

Adhesive Technology for
Restorative Dentistry

Edited by

Jean-François Roulet, DDS, Dr Med Dent, PhD

Professor and Director
Department of Operative and Preventive Dentistry and Endodontics
School of Dental Medicine
Charité—Universitätsmedizin Berlin
Campus Virchow Clinic
Berlin, Germany

Guido Vanherle, MD, DDS

Emeritus Professor
Department of Operative Dentistry and Dental Materials
School of Dentistry, Oral Pathology, and Maxillofacial Surgery
Faculty of Medicine
Catholic University of Leuven
Leuven, Belgium

Quintessence Publishing Co, Ltd
London, Chicago, Berlin, Tokyo, Paris, Milan, Barcelona, Istanbul, São Paulo, New Delhi, Moscow, Prague and Warsaw

British Library Catalouging in Publication Data

European Symposium on Adhesive Dentistry (3rd: 2001: Berlin, Germany)
Adhesive technology for restorative dentistry
1. Dental adhesives – Congresses 2. Dentistry, Operative – Congresses
I. Title II. Roulet, Jean-Francois III. Vanherle, Guido
617.6'95

ISBN 1850971072
Printed in Germany

© 2005 Quintessence Publishing Co, Ltd

Quintessence Publishing Co, Ltd
Grafton Road
New Malden
London, Surrey
KT3 3AB
United Kingdom
www.quintpub.co.uk

Table of Contents

Preface

Another book on adhesive dentistry? Is there a need for it? We asked ourselves these questions when deciding whether to compile the proceedings from the 3rd European Symposium on Adhesive Dentistry, held in Berlin in September 2001. We came to the clear conclusion that, yes, this information needed to be published, despite the fact that adhesive techniques have already penetrated almost all fields of practiced dentistry. Adhesive techniques have become very complex, and many factors must be considered with each specific clinical application.

In addition, there is still a gap between accepted treatment modes in adhesive dentistry and what is carried out in daily practice. Although new methods are beneficial for the dentition, changes in delivery of care are progressing at a slow pace. While researchers and academics are pushing the frontiers of adhesive dentistry well into acceptable limits for clinical practice, practitioners hesitate to change. They need more information, more arguments, and more data before making a decision. An attempt is made in this book to facilitate decisions and changes in the right direction.

The book can be divided into four sections. In chapters 1 through 3, leaders in the field present rationale for adhesive techniques in esthetic restorative dentistry. Chapters 4 through 7 deal with minimally invasive dentistry, which is possible only because of advances in adhesive technology. Chapters 8 through 10 are devoted to specific issues a clinician will face when using adhesive techniques with ceramic and resin composite restorations. Finally, chapters 11 and 12 remind us that we are not "adhesive technocrats" but dentists operating in a biologic system with the objective to restore the health of our patients.

In closing, we must thank all the authors for their contributions and the GC Corporation, whose generous sponsorship made the symposium possible.

Jean-François Roulet
Guido Vanherle

Contributors

Aylin Baysan, BDS, MSc, PhD
Clinical Lecturer
Department of Restorative Dentistry
School of Dentistry
University of Birmingham
Birmingham, United Kingdom

Marc Braem, DDS, PhD, FADM
Professor
Lab Dental Materials
University of Antwerp
Antwerp, Belgium

F. J. Trevor Burke, DDS, MSc, MDS
Professor of Primary Dental Care
School of Dentistry
University of Birmingham
Birmingham, United Kingdom

Garry J. P. Fleming, BSc, PhD
Lecturer in Biomaterials
School of Dentistry
University of Birmingham
Birmingham, United Kingdom

Galip Gürel, DDS, MSc
Private Practice
Istanbul, Turkey

Paul Lambrechts, DDS, Dr Med Dent, PhD, Prof Dr Dent
Professor
Department of Dentistry and
  Maxillofacial Surgery
School of Dentistry, Oral Pathology, and
  Maxillofacial Surgery
Faculty of Medicine
Catholic University of Leuven
Leuven, Belgium

Götz M. Lösche, Dr Med Dent
Assistant Professor
Department of Operative and
  Preventive Dentistry and Endodontics
School of Dental Medicine
Charité—Universitätsmedizin Berlin
Campus Virchow Clinic
Berlin, Germany

Edward Lynch, BDentSc, MA, FDSRCSEd, PhD
Professor
Department of Restorative Dentistry and
  Gerodontology
Queen's University Belfast
Belfast, Northern Ireland

Peter M. Marquis, BSc, PhD
Professor of Biomaterials
Director and Head of School
School of Dentistry
University of Birmingham
Birmingham, United Kingdom

Ivar A. Mjör, BDS, MSD, MS, Dr Odont
Professor and Eminent Scholar
Department of Operative Dentistry
College of Dentistry
University of Florida
Gainesville, Florida

Graham J. Mount, AM, BDS, DDSc
Visiting Research Fellow
University of Adelaide
Adelaide, South Australia

Dan Nathanson, DDS
Professor and Chair
Department of Restorative
  Sciences/Biomaterials
Goldman School of Dental Medicine
Boston University
Boston, Massachusetts

Marleen Peumans, DDS, PhD
Clinical Instructor and Research Associate
Department of Operative Dentistry and
  Dental Materials
School of Dentistry, Oral Pathology, and
  Maxillofacial Surgery
Faculty of Medicine
Catholic University of Leuven
Leuven, Belgium

**Jean-François Roulet, DDS,
Dr Med Dent, PhD**
Professor and Director
Department of Operative and Preventive
  Dentistry and Endodontics
School of Dental Medicine
Charité—Universitätsmedizin Berlin
Campus Virchow Clinic
Berlin, Germany

Roberto Spreafico, DMD
Private Practice
Busto-Arsizio, Italy

Jan W. V. van Dijken, Dr Odont, DDS, PhD
Professor
Department of Odontology
Dental School Umeå
Umeå University
Umeå, Sweden

Bart Van Meerbeek, DDS, PhD
Professor
Leuven BIOMAT Research Cluster
Department of Conservative Dentistry
School of Dentistry, Oral Pathology, and
  Maxillofacial Surgery
Faculty of Medicine
Catholic University of Leuven
Leuven, Belgium

Richard van Noort, BSc, DPhil
Professor and Head of Department
Department of Adult Dental Care
University of Sheffield
Sheffield, United Kingdom

Guido Vanherle, MD, DDS
Emeritus Professor
Department of Operative Dentistry and
  Dental Materials
School of Dentistry, Oral Pathology, and
  Maxillofacial Surgery
Faculty of Medicine
Catholic University of Leuven
Leuven, Belgium

**Stefan Zimmer, DDS, Dr Med Dent,
PhD**
Associate Professor
Department of Operative and Preventive
  Dentistry and Endodontics
Heinrich Heine University
Düsseldorf, Germany

Chapter 1

How Important Are Esthetics?

Guido Vanherle, Marleen Peumans,
Bart Van Meerbeek, Paul Lambrechts

Abstract

Caries incidence has been reduced in Western societies. Thanks to improved preventive measures, fewer and smaller carious lesions are being seen. Periodontal health can be assured if the patient's commitment to oral hygiene can be obtained. Extensive restorative treatments are less frequent, and patients are now retaining their teeth longer than in previous generations. As a result, other needs are emerging. The advent and development of adhesive dentistry have changed treatment modalities considerably. The direct adhesive use of tooth-colored restorative materials has opened new opportunities. Improved dental esthetics are now affordable for a wide range of patients. When basic requirements for caries control, periodontal health, and masticatory function are met in the dentition, proven and safe clinical techniques to enhance esthetics should be considered for treatment of serious esthetic deficiencies. Careful planning and postoperative follow-up are necessary to guarantee the enduring success of that intervention. Esthetic treatments are therefore indicated when esthetic dysfunctions exist, when a feasible therapeutic approach is available, and when both the patient and clinician agree on the proposed outcome.

It has long been realized that the restoration of traumatic or extensive carious lesions in the anterior dentition has an impact on the appearance of the patient. Therefore, such restorations are very demanding because the clinician must not only treat the lesion or the defect but also restore esthetics, which is one of the social functions of our dentition.

The most important function of our dentition is mastication. All human beings must acquire and maintain the ability to bring food into the oral cavity and prepare it for further digestion and assimilation into the body. A normal dentition is a prerequisite for good masticatory function.

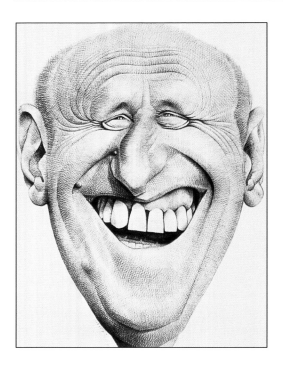

Fig 1-1 Nature has harmoniously combined form and tooth position with the peculiarities of this face.

The dentition also plays an important role in the maintenance of other functions, such as phonation and social exchanges. Especially for the latter, the mineralized and hard tissues of the dentition, together with the maxilla and mandible, support the soft tissues of the subnasal part of the face. Here, the dentition has a direct impact on the facial morphology of the individual. While the morphologic characteristics of the lower part of the human face are determined primarily by the bony structures of the maxilla and mandible, in normal social contacts the dentition is the most visible factor.

Undeniably, the dentition plays an important role in one's appearance, as one's facial image is largely determined by the color, morphology, and position of the teeth.[1]

The Esthetic Function of the Dentition

In every social contact, an individual is perceived and judged by the expression on his or her face, which becomes the focus of one's attention. In every encounter, one would like to explore the exact nature of that other person.[1] What are his or her feelings and intentions? What is his or her character like? The eyes and the mouth are the first to attract attention, as they express the character of the person one is encountering.[2] In most cases, a gentle smile will disclose the front teeth and either improve or disturb the harmony of the face.

The importance of the dentition in facial expression is demonstrated in Fig 1-1, in which the dentition is in perfect harmony with the face of this ever-joking French comedian. Nature has done a wonderful job here in combining form and position harmoniously with the peculiarities of his face and his overall personality.

Characteristics such as health, well-being, a sense of order, and discipline will find important expression in the human dentition as in all other parts of the body.[1] Very often this is defined as perfect harmony or esthetic appearance. What is esthetics? A dictionary defines it as follows: "Esthetics is everything that can provoke a perception of beauty." Thus, esthetics is very often a personal or a common appreciation. Appreciation and perception of beauty varies in different ethnic populations and also throughout historical periods. Today, in most parts of the world, a normal and healthy dentition is an absolute prerequisite for a pleasing and esthetic appearance.[3] Clinicians cannot afford to ignore this simple fact of life. But there is still a question: How far do we have to go to obtain an esthetic dentition?

The Evolution of Dental Care

Historically, and even today in certain parts of the world, dental care is restricted to the alleviation of pain and discomfort. With the introduction of restorative materials in dentistry, carious lesions were treated, and the teeth were retained in spite of the limitations of these restorative materials. Large cavities had to be drilled and sound tissue sacrificed to create the retentive conditions for a long-lasting result. Because of these interventions, millions of teeth could be saved, and normal oral function could continue for many years. However, that treatment, which aimed to stop the infection and the pain, also had its disadvantages. The initial lesion frequently recurred because no adequate remedy was available to combat leakage and cariogenic flora. Furthermore, the gradual breakdown of the restored teeth, which resulted from the loss of tissue, was one of the consequences of such restorative care.

Adhesive dentistry eliminates some of the drawbacks of conventional restorative dentistry. New materials were proposed and new methods tested.[4] It took more than 40 years to reach an acceptable level of confidence. It all started with the restoration of fractured incisal edges.[5] Enamel etching, initially scorned by colleagues in the profession, proved to be a reasonable method to enable restorative material to bond to fractured anterior teeth, especially in younger patients for whom a prosthetic solution had to be postponed for biologic reasons.[6] That therapy quickly became a success story all over the world and opened the door for more change[7,8] (Figs 1-2a and 1-2b).

Shortly thereafter orthodontists realized the advantages of bonding brackets directly to enamel, thus eliminating the need for multiple bands. Orthodontic therapy became easier and more affordable.

Some time later clinicians started to use enamel bonding to restore small carious lesions in anterior teeth.[9] Pushing this new technique to its limits, they achieved invisible restorations (Figs 1-3a and 1-3b), which could be perceived only by a well-trained eye.

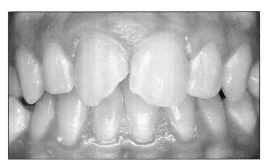

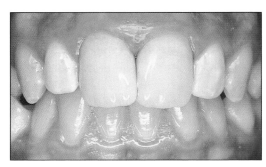

Fig 1-2a Fractured central incisors before treatment.

Fig 1-2b Appearance of the incisors after treatment.

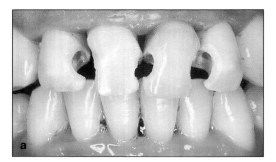

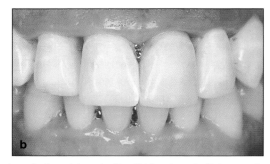

Figs 1-3a and 1-3b Several Class III and Class IV lesions before (a) and after (b) treatment. Only a well-trained eye can detect a dental intervention. These restorations are truly esthetic.

Dental adhesive techniques also simplified the immediate and definitive treatment of traumatic injuries.[5] It took many years to change the prevailing beliefs of the profession, as textbooks continued to advocate the classic preparations for conventional nonadhesive materials.

In the 1980s, enamel bonding became generally accepted in the profession both by academics and by general practitioners. The most progressive practitioners again pushed the limits. Diastemata, often unresolved by orthodontists because of a tooth-arch discrepancy, could easily be handled with a reversible treatment using enamel bonding and direct restorative materials[10] (Figs 1-4a and

1-4b). The change of tooth form through the addition of direct restorative materials was a breakthrough in restorative dentistry because it eliminated the need for crowns or the irreversible sacrifice of more tooth tissue.[11–13]

It became apparent that adhesive dentistry had crossed a point of no return: A pleasing appearance could be created with a minimum amount of restorative materials and a minimum number of instruments. Investigations proved the benefits of such treatments,[14] and although the durability of these restorations was inferior to the classic fixed partial denture, they were definitely less traumatic and less expensive.[15]

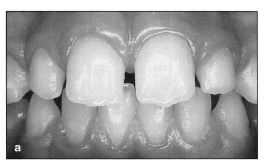
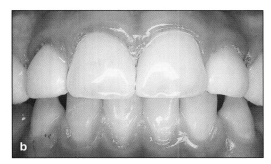

Figs 1-4a and 1-4b Diastemata due to a tooth-arch discrepancy before treatment *(a)*, and after treatment *(b)*. Tooth form, alignment, the golden proportion, and the midline have been respected.

Greater difficulties were encountered when bonding to dentin, and only recently have techniques and materials been developed to offer comparable results to enamel bonding.[16] Nowadays, this problem seems to have been largely resolved.[17,18] As patients keep their teeth longer, cervical lesions are becoming more frequent, with dentin as the only substrate to be bonded to.[19,20] The circular root lesions often present in older teeth are difficult to manage without adhesive dentistry.

Clinical investigations have demonstrated the feasibility of adhesive restorative dentistry,[8,21] and efficient preventive measures have proved to counteract the impact of caries on the human dentition. Smaller and fewer lesions are encountered today.[22,23] Studies have shown that microorganisms cannot survive in a sealed restoration, so caries progression underneath these restorations is stopped.[24] With reduced caries occurrence and more restorative possibilities, treatment requirements have shifted.[25] Pain is no longer the principal motive for a dental appointment. Other needs are emerging, while the older ones are diminishing and newer possibilities are becoming available.

Changing Life Patterns

In the Western world, the media is often the predominant source of information, and its influence extends around the world. From dawn to dusk, information pours out in different forms and formulas, and it is always accompanied by advertising. The most striking theme in advertising is that "beautiful is always better." This is especially characteristic among salespeople, people in the public sector, and actors, who in their daily work have to please as many people as possible. Their appearance is therefore very important.[26]

Not every human being is born with a pleasing appearance, so plastic surgery, dermatologic intervention, and dental treatment are often needed to satisfy the minimum requirements of social contact.[27] These treatments or interventions are focused not only on improving appearance but also on enhancing interaction with others. In a highly competitive world, a pleasing appearance is often the difference between success and failure.[28]

The role of dentistry in providing an acceptable appearance cannot be ignored, and although most practitioners are trained to relieve pain and maintain the masticatory function of the dentition, they should not forget that other functions are also important. While it is right to focus on the lifetime function of the dentition, as this is its principal purpose, other treatments that improve esthetics and clearly benefit the individual without harming the dentition or other oral structures must not be excluded. When the principal requirements are met, esthetic demands must be heard, analyzed, and addressed in a justified manner. Although an unpleasing color is not a disease per se, the patient may consider it a disease, meaning that the oral condition disturbs his or her well-being.

Conditions and Rules for Esthetic Treatments

Clinical investigations are still needed to set the limits of current restorative materials and techniques.[29] In the last three or four decades, tooth-colored materials have been subject to scrutiny all over the world. For the restoration of anterior teeth, resin composites maintain their lead, but other materials available on the market also have their advantages. Microfilled resin composites can offer improved esthetics but are vulnerable in stress-bearing locations.[30–32] Small-particle hybrids or medium-filled, densified composites also offer more strength and

acceptable esthetics,[33] and they are the materials of choice in larger restorations. Ultrafine, compact-filled, densified composites are the materials of choice in the posterior region because they combine strength, wear resistance, and surface smoothness.[34]

Enamel and dentin bonding have gained widespread acceptance, and long-term clinical results indicate that the best results can be obtained using smear-layer removal systems in a total-etch form applied in three steps.[17] New materials with a reduced application time and less risk of error are still under investigation.[35] A sealed restoration has definite advantages over a conventional restoration with no bonding. This is particularly true for small restorations or restorations where sufficient tooth structure is present to counteract the shrinkage stresses induced during the curing of the resin composites.

Bonded resin composite restorations are less durable than metallic and porcelain structures, but the invasive and irreversible character of an indirect approach offsets much of their advantage. Last but not least, their cost makes them unaffordable for much of the population.[36]

Bonded restorations can last for more than 5 years if patients maintain an acceptable level of oral hygiene, and minor adjustments can extend this time.[13] The periodontal response is acceptable as long as fundamental rules are respected.[13,37–39]

Today many lesions can be treated with a direct method. Sometimes, this approach can be used as a temporary solution in anticipation of more complicated work (Figs 1-5a and 1-5b). A re-

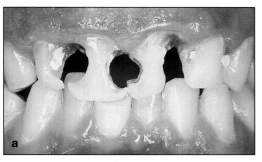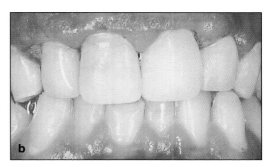

Figs 1-5a and 1-5b Severe and minor defects on the central and lateral incisors *(a)*. A direct adhesive restorative treatment *(b)* has resulted in an acceptable temporary solution in anticipation of more complicated work.

versible treatment mode will provide the clinician with time to prepare a more complex intervention. Nevertheless, all direct restorations need a minimum amount of dental substrate for bonding. If the amount available is insufficient, an indirect approach must be considered.

How far should practitioners go to enhance esthetics? The answer is, as far as the dental treatment remains a treatment. Nowadays, the proper use of resin composites with adhesive techniques is entirely justified in the anterior dentition and partially justified in the posterior region.[40] Nevertheless, all treatment must be based on sound professional judgment and not on experimentation or on emotional or financial motives.

All treatment must be based on the basic rules of dental care. First, normal function of the dentition must be guaranteed over the long term.[41] Second, all harm must be excluded.

Therefore, all carious lesions must be eliminated first, the pulp tissue must be allowed to recover, and then the defects have to be repaired. That process will take some time, so the clinician will have

an opportunity to develop a plan for addressing other requirements. All caries activity must be reduced to a normal level by means of normal or additional caries-preventive measures. The outcome of this approach can also be measured. Oral hygiene must be sufficient so that periodontal health can be assured. Monitoring the patient over long periods is necessary. Finally, all treatments must result in acceptable masticatory function. Once these basic requirements are met, the esthetic treatment can be considered, as it can enhance the benefit of the overall treatment and increase the satisfaction of both the patient and the practitioner.

Patients can exhibit different levels of oral fitness. Those who can meet the basic requirements concerning caries activity, periodontal health, and masticatory function over long periods of time can be considered for esthetic treatment. Others must participate in a series of preliminary sessions that provide information about not smoking or eating or drinking substances that may harm the restorations before they can become a candidate for esthetic treatment. Clinicians have to be flexible in their daily work but should not forget that a number of patients are orally unfit for esthetic restorations. The basic rules for success in dentistry must not be neglected, because esthetic restorative dentistry can be a minefield for the clinician. Commitment from both the patient and the dentist is needed to ensure long-term success. In cases where this is lacking, it is wiser to refrain from acting.

As dental esthetic restorations are judged by the final outcome rather than by the effort invested in realizing them, careful attention should be paid to the preparation of the treatment. Clinicians must have a clear knowledge of the prospects offered by esthetic interventions. Furthermore, the practitioner has to know the results of controlled clinical investigations, which provide information about the longevity of these treatments. Each new clinical technique should undergo validation against objective criteria over a long period of time and in sufficient numbers so that the limits of application can be clearly designated. Within the established limits, a particular restoration mode can be justified.

Practitioners must not only be familiar with the different esthetic dysfunctions that can occur in the dentition,[42] they must also be able to grade them on a scale from minor to severe. Treatment, if affordable, should be advocated when the dysfunction is clearly disturbing. In such cases, both the patient and the clinician must have a say in the decision making.

Patients with esthetic complaints often make demands beyond the clinician's ability to treat the situation, and some-times patients are unable to define the dysfunction of their appearance. Therefore, a careful discussion, perhaps aided by study casts and photographs, should precede all treatment.[43] Patients who opt for a direct approach using resin composite materials must be aware of certain obligations afterward. In addition to rigorous oral hygiene, they must refrain from consuming food or drinks rich in pigments. For the same reason, smoking should be ceased. Finally, an annual visit to the practitioner is needed to assess and possibly repair shortcomings. Although esthetics are not essential for the survival of the dentition, their careful selection and application will provide great satisfaction and function to the patient.

Conclusion

As the incidence of caries has been reduced and patients keep their teeth longer, patients are requesting more treatment to enhance esthetics. The advent of adhesive dentistry and the development of resin composites have opened new possibilities for dental esthetics. With careful selection of an adhesive technique by the clinician and diligent oral hygiene by the patient, bonded composite restorations can provide a successful outcome that satisfies the requirements of both parties.

References

1. Rufenacht CR. Fundamentals of Esthetics. Chicago: Quintessence, 1992.

2. Baldwin DC. Appearance and esthetics in oral health. Community Dent Oral Epidemiol 1980; 8:224–256.

3. Qualtrough AJE, Burke FJT. A look at dental esthetics. Quintessence Int 1994;25:7–14.

4. Ferracane JL. Current trends in dental composites. Crit Rev Oral Biol Med 1995;6:302–318.

5. Andreasen J. Adhesive dentistry applied to the treatment of traumatic dental injuries. Oper Dent 2001;26:328–335.

6. Ward GT, Buonocore MG, Woolridge ED Jr. Preliminary report of a technique using Nuva-Seal in the treatment and repair of anterior fractures without pins. N Y State Dent J 1972;38: 269–274.

7. Andreasen FM, Andreasen JO. Crown fractures. In: Andreasen JO, Andreasen FM (eds). Textbook and Colour Atlas of Traumatic Injuries in the Teeth. Copenhagen: Munksgaard, 1994: 219–250.

8. Smales RJ. Effects of enamel-bonding, type of restoration, patient age and operator on the longevity of an anterior composite resin. Am J Dent 1991;4:130–133.

9. Porte A, Lutz F, Lund MR, Swartz ML, Cochran MA. Cavity designs for composite resins. Oper Dent 1984;9:50–56.

10. Albers HF. Direct composite veneers. In: Bonded Tooth-Colored Restoratives, ed 7. Santa Rosa, CA: Alto Books, 1985:7-1–7-32.

11. Black JB. Esthetic restoration of tetracycline-stained teeth. J Am Dent Assoc 1982;104: 846–851.

12. Calamia JR. Etched porcelain veneers: The current state of the art. Quintessence Int 1985; 1:5–12.

13. Peumans M. The clinical performance of veneer restorations and their influence on the periodontium [thesis]. Leuven, Belgium: Leuven University Press, 1997.

14. Peumans M, Van Meerbeek B, Lambrechts P, Vanherle G. The 5-year clinical performance of direct composite additions to correct tooth form and position. I: Esthetic qualities. Clin Oral Investig 1997;1:12–18.

15. Peumans M, Van Meerbeek B, Lambrechts P, Vanherle G. The 5-year clinical performance of direct composite additions to correct tooth form and position. II. Marginal Qualities. Clin Oral Investig 1997;1:19–26.

16. Van Meerbeek B, Perdigão J, Lambrechts P, Vanherle G. The clinical performance of adhesives. J Dent 1998;26:1–20.

17. Van Meerbeek B, Peumans M, Gladys S, Braem M, Lambrechts P, Vanherle G. Three-year clinical effectiveness of four total-etch dentinal adhesive systems in cervical lesions. Quintessence Int 1996;27:775–784.

18. Van Meerbeek B, Peumans M, Verschueren M, et al. Clinical status of ten dentin adhesive systems. J Dent Res 1994;73:1690–1702.

19. Van Meerbeek B, Braem M, Lambrechts P, Vanherle G. Morphological characterization of the interface between resin and sclerotic dentine. J Dent 1994;22:141–146.

20. Vanherle G, Lambrechts P, Braem M. An evaluation of different adhesive restorations in cervical lesions. J Prosthet Dent 1991;65:341–347.

21. Smales RJ. Long-term deterioration of composite resin and amalgam restorations. Oper Dent 1991;16:202–209.

22. Cahen PM, Turlot JC, Clement G, Seckler G. Comparative study of oral conditions in schoolchildren of Strasbourg. Community Dent Oral Epidemiol 1987;15:211–215.

23. Marthaler TM, O'Mullane DM, Vrbic V. The prevalence of dental caries in Europe. Caries Res 1996;30:237–255.

24. Mertz-Fairhurst EJ, Curtis JW Jr, Ergle JW, Rueggeberg FA, Adair SM. Ultraconservative and cariostatic sealed restorations: Results at year 10. J Am Dent Assoc 1998;129:55–66.

25. Reinhardt JW, Capiulouto ML. Composite resin esthetic dentistry survey in New England. J Am Dent Assoc 1990;120:541–544.

26. Jenny J, Proshek JM. Visibility and prestige of occupations and the importance of dental appearance. J Can Dent Assoc 1986;12:987–989.

27. Davis LG, Ashworth PD, Spriggs LS. Psychological effects of aesthetic dental treatment. J Dent 1998;26:547–554.

28. Linn EL. Social meaning of dental appearance. J Health Hum Behav 1966;7:295–298.

29. Lambrechts P. Basic properties of dental composites and their impact on clinical performance [thesis]. Leuven, Belgium: Acco, 1983.

30. Lambrechts P, Ameye C, Vanherle G. Conventional and microfilled composite resin. Part II: Chip factures. J Prosthet Dent 1982;48:527–538.

31. Willems G, Lambrechts P, Braem M, Celis JP, Vanherle G. A classification of dental composites according to their morphological and mechanical characteristics. Dent Mater 1992;8:310–319.

32. Willems G, Lambrechts P, Braem M, Vanherle G. Composite resins in the 21st century. Quintessence Int 1993;24:641–658.

33. Peumans M, Willems G, Lambrechts P, Braem M, Vanherle G. Structure of anterior composites related to their clinical behavior [abstract 100]. J Dent Res 1989;68:621.

34. Willems G, Lambrechts P, Braem M, Vanherle G. Three-year follow-up of five posterior composites: In vivo wear. J Dent 1993;21:74–78.

35. Van Meerbeek B, Vargas M, Inoue S, et al. Adhesives and cements to promote preservation dentistry. Oper Dent 2001;suppl 6:119–144.

36. Goldstein RE, Lancaster JS. Survey of patient attitudes toward current esthetic procedures. J Prosthet Dent 1984;52:775–780.

37. Blank LW, Caffesse RG, Charbeneau GT. The gingival response of well-finished composite resin restorations. J Am Dent Assoc 1979;42:626–632.

38. Blank LW, Caffesse RG, Charbeneau GT. The gingival response of well-finished composite resin restorations. A 28-month report. J Prosthet Dent 1981;46:157–160.

39. Peumans M, Van Meerbeek B, Lambrechts P, Vanherle G, Quirynen M. The influence of direct composite additions for the correction of tooth form and/or position on periodontal health. A retrospective study. J Periodontol 1998;69: 422–427.

40. Smith DC. General discussion. In: Vanherle G, Degrange M, Willems G (eds). State of the Art on Direct Posterior Filling Materials and Dentine Bonding. Leuven, Belgium: Van der Poorten, 1993:251–269.

41. Guichet DL, Guichet NF. From function to esthetics: Anterior or occlusal compromises to esthetics. Curr Opin Cosmet Dent 1993:55–60.

42. Albers HF. Esthetic treatment planning. Adept Report 1992;3:45–52.

43. Levine JB. Esthetic diagnosis. Curr Opin Cosmet Dent 1995:9–17.

Chapter 2

Composite Layering

Roberto Spreafico, Jean-François Roulet

Abstract

Composite layering allows the clinician to accomplish invisible restorations—that is, restorations that cannot be perceived by the patient. The prerequisite is the meticulous application of adhesive technology and the use of composite materials in different translucencies: "dentin," "enamel," and special effect material (eg, "clear"). Using these materials, dentin is replaced by an opaque composite and enamel by a more translucent one to mimic nature. Furthermore, mechanical and physical properties must be respected, especially in large and complex cavities. For these cases, a special layering technique is proposed for restoration of both anterior and posterior teeth. In the anterior segment there are two options: Many cases can be satisfactorily restored with a two-layer technique, or a three-layer technique can be used to obtain the best esthetic integration of the restoration.

Esthetic dentistry requires the clinician to mimic the natural tooth by inserting restorations that are invisible (or at least imperceptible) to the patient. To do so, the clinician must be familiar with the neighboring structures, such as the tooth to be restored, adjacent teeth, the antagonists, the lips, and the whole face. The less structure that remains, the more the reconstruction is guided by the knowledge of esthetics—rules that govern shapes, proportions, relations, and colors.[1,2] This is the case if complete dentures or extensive fixed partial denture reconstructions are fabricated. In operative dentistry there is usually a different challenge: Only portions of a single tooth are to be reconstructed. Therefore, the different anatomic structures of the single

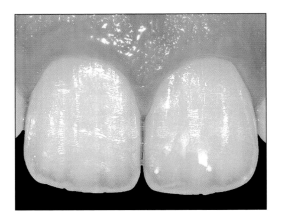

Fig 2-1 Natural incisors of a young individual. Note the transparent areas in the incisal region, the microstructure of the surface, the yellowish shining of the incisal edge, and the small notches in the incisal edge.

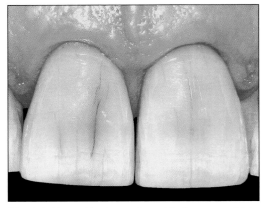

Fig 2-2 Natural incisors of an elderly person. Note the signs of wear and stress (eg, cracks).

tooth or the adjacent teeth become very important. In this case, the objective is to imitate existing tooth structures as accurately as possible (Figs 2-1 and 2-2), which is possible with small-particle hybrid composite materials.

There are three prerequisites to achieve invisible restorations: *(1)* perfect integration of the restorative material with the tooth tissue by excellent adhesion[3–6]; *(2)* the use of resin composite of different opacities ("enamel," "dentin," and effects, eg, "clear") with a layering technique to obtain perfect color match; and *(3)* perfect integration of the form and macro- and microsurface texture of the composite restoration with the remaining natural surface.

Rationale for Layering

Layering is the superimposition of various increments of composite material light-cured separately. The technique is performed for a variety of reasons.

Minimize Polymerization Stresses

Today's composite materials are polymerized with a free-radical polymerization, which inherently leads to shrinkage of the material while monomers are converted into a polymer. With intelligent resin selection and optimal filling of the material with a multitude of fillers, this shrinkage could be reduced but not suppressed.[7] Shrinkage means a volume loss of the composite in the cavity. If the material is bonded to the cavity walls, as it is with adhesive techniques, the interface will be subjected to stress.[8] Several factors contribute to the polymerization stresses: material composition (resin, filler type, and load), modulus of elasticity of the composite, degree of polymerization, speed of polymerization, composite volume, and restoration geometry (c-factor). Because they are all interrelated,[9] controlling polymerization stress is very difficult. Layering is one option to reduce this stress, because small

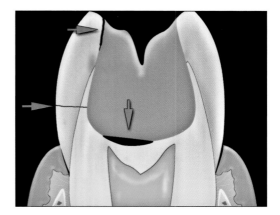

Fig 2-3 Consequences of polymerization stresses on large posterior cavities are marginal openings, internal debonding, cuspal flexure, and even cusp fractures.

increments placed in a preparation with an intelligent geometry produce less stress.

With bulk techniques, independent of all other factors, more stresses are imposed, causing negative consequences (Fig 2-3), such as marginal openings, internal debondings, cuspal flexure, and cusp microfractures.

Increase Polymerization Depth

The curing light is absorbed and dispersed by the composite material. Therefore, the degree of curing is a function of depth (distance from the surface, where the light tip is applied). Usually 2 to 3 mm is considered a safe curing depth, if the curing light is working properly and is not absorbed by tooth structures.[10,11] Layering enables the dentist to build up large restorations without sacrificing the degree of curing and thus mechanical properties in deep layers.

Achieve Accurate Anatomic Contour

It is much easier to achieve a natural-looking anatomy with an additive technique (layering the uncured material) than with a subtractive technique (grinding the cured composite).

Obtain Optimal Esthetics

With any layering technique an optimal esthetic outcome can be expected if two principles are followed:

1. Replace dentin with opaque composite and replace enamel with transparent composite.
2. By creating a bevel, the transition between the tooth color and the composite color is not precisely defined. With this technique, the eye is deceived, because it is excellent at detecting sharp contrast but only fair at realizing smooth transitions from one color nuance into another.

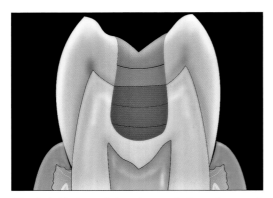

Fig 2-4 Horizontal layering technique for small cavities.

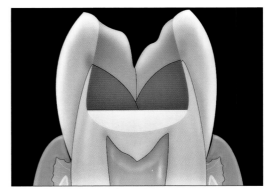

Fig 2-5 Diagonal layering technique for medium-sized cavities.

Layering Techniques for Posterior Teeth

Small Cavities

For small cavities it is easiest to perform a horizontal layering technique (Fig 2-4). After caries has been removed, the dentin is perfectly sealed by careful application of the bonding system. It is very important to completely cure the bonding layer before the first increment of composite is placed. With this measure, a complete sealing of the dentin is obtained by hybridization,[12] which aids in preventing postoperative sensitivity. Clinical experience has shown that if the first increment is placed with a flowable composite, postoperative sensitivity can be completely eliminated. This may be due to the lower modulus of elasticity of flowable composites. This layer is then able to absorb some of the polymerization stresses from the subsequent layers without inducing stress on the adhesive-dentin interface (in this way it acts as a gasket). According to the hydrodynamic theory for postoperative pain as explained by Brännström et al,[13,14] postop-

erative pain is generated by fluid movements that occur within the dentinal tubules if voids are formed between the restoration and the dentin.

The subsequent layers are then placed with an opaque "dentin" composite. For most cases the color A3 or A3.5 is used. Then a final transparent "enamel" composite layer is placed and well-adapted to the cavity walls prior to curing. If a glycerin gel (eg, Airblock, Dentsply, Konstant, Germany; or Liquistrip, Ivoclar Vivadent, Schaan, Lichtenstein) is placed before the final curing, the oxygen inhibition layer will not form.[15] The benefit of this technique is that it requires minimal finishing and polishing.

Medium-sized Cavities

For medium-sized cavities, a diagonal layering technique (Fig 2-5) is superior because it takes advantage of a more favorable c-factor.[16] As in the small cavity, a meticulous adhesive technique is very important. Note that when the dentin masses are applied, they must be kept short of the finishing line so that space is maintained for the enamel masses. Simultaneously with the applica-

Fig 2-6 Mid-sized Class I cavity restored with the diagonal layering technique.

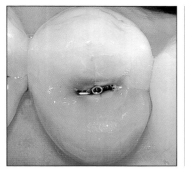

Fig 2-6a The carious lesion.

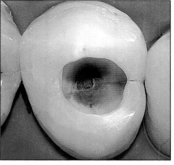

Fig 2-6b The decayed tissue is removed and the etching completed.

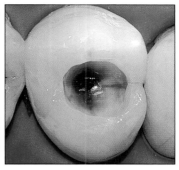

Fig 2-6c The bonding procedure is completed with careful light curing.

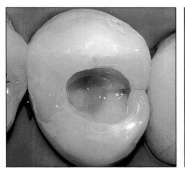

Fig 2-6d The first layer is placed with a flowable composite.

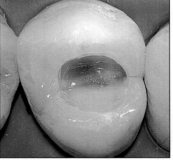

Fig 2-6e The palatal dentin increment is placed. Note that it must stay approximally 1 mm short of the finishing line.

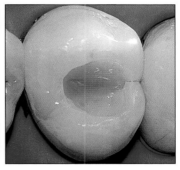

Fig 2-6f The buccal increment is placed and formed according to the anatomy.

Figs 2-6g and 2-6h The enamel layer is placed and the fissure characterized with intensive stain.

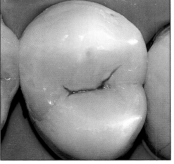

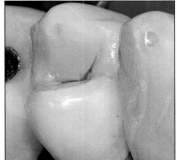

tion of the enamel masses, in the depth of the fissures, minute amounts of intensive stain (eg, Kolor Plus brown, SDS Kerr, Orange, CA; or Tetric Color, dunkelbraun, Ivoclar Vivadent, Schaan, Lichtenstein) may be placed (Fig 2-6).

Fig 2-7 Class II composite restoration.

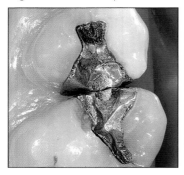 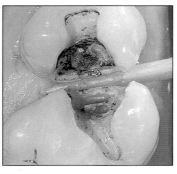 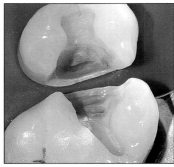

Fig 2-7a Old, defective amalgam restorations that must be replaced.

Fig 2-7b Amalgams are removed without enlarging the cavity size. Note the oxides still present on the cavity walls. The wooden wedge is placed to displace the papilla and prevent it from being damaged by the preparation diamonds.

Fig 2-7c Finished cavity preparations.

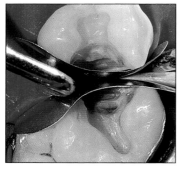 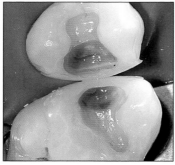 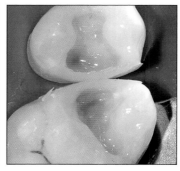

Fig 2-7d The sectional matrix bands are placed. The clamp is separating the teeth slightly. It is very important to check the cervical adaptation of the matrix bands. It must be perfect to avoid overhangs.

Fig 2-7e After the bonding system has been applied and cured, the proximal walls are built up in one increment against the matrix bands, taking advantage of the c-factor.

Fig 2-7f The cavity is "lined" with a thin layer of flowable composite.

Class II composite restorations are a challenge for the clinician for many reasons. Because composite cannot be condensed as amalgam can, it is difficult to achieve a tight contact point, especially if circular matrix bands are used. With these bands, the proximal anatomy is usually not correct, because the bands do not sufficiently imitate the convex shape of the tooth crown. This results in a weak contact point as well as one that is placed too far occlusally. Once cured, excess material is difficult to remove without damaging hard tooth substance.

Due to an unfavorable c-factor and maybe poor enamel quality cervically,

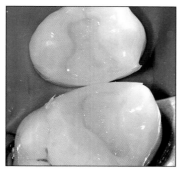

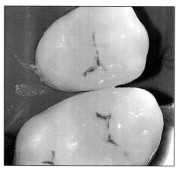

Fig 2-7g The dentin composite is placed, following the contour of the final anatomy but 1 mm short of the margins.

Fig 2-7h Stain is placed in the grooves, and the final anatomy is developed with enamel composite.

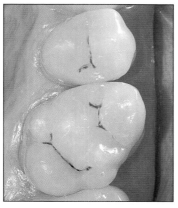

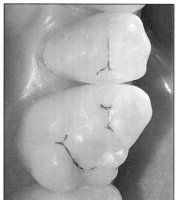

Fig 2-7i Restorations immediately after placement.

Fig 2-7j Restorations after 12 months in service.

Class II restorations show a poor margin quality, especially in the proximal and cervical areas. In this case, a special layering technique using preformed, sectional metal matrix bands (Palodent, Dentsply Caulk, Konstant, Germany) together with a separating clamp and taking advantage of the c-factor has proven to be successful both experimentally[17] and clinically (Fig 2-7). With this technique, after the bonding system is applied and cured, the proximal walls are built up in one increment against the matrix bands. This relies heavily on the principles of the c-factor; because the composite does not adhere to the matrix band and has a large surface facing the

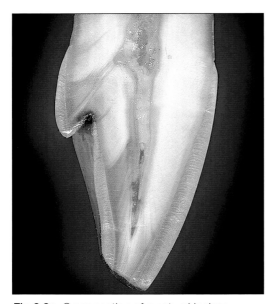

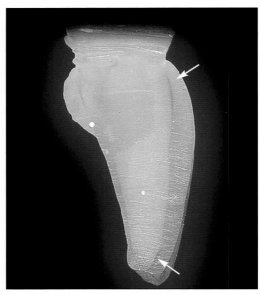

Fig 2-8a Cross section of a natural incisor.

Fig 2-8b Composite incisor consisting of two enamel layers and one dentin core made with two different shades. For special effects, intensive stain was used, as always, *under* the enamel layer (arrows).

open box, the free surface is very large. From both of these surfaces the composite can compensate for the shrinkage until the gel point is reached without building up stress at the small bonded surfaces (cervical and axial). After polymerization, which must be done carefully to prevent shadows from the metal matrix band, the matrix system is removed. Now the Class II situation is converted into a Class I and can be restored as previously described.

Anterior Teeth: Superior Techniques with Layering

In the anterior segment, layering helps to achieve the "invisible" restoration. As a rule, one tries to imitate with the composite material the same layers nature has created (Fig 2-8). This would indicate the need for a three-layer technique. However, especially with opaque teeth, there may be insufficient space to place dentin material between the two enamel layers, which would result in a restoration that appears too dark, or *too transparent*. In these cases, a two-layer technique is used, in which the palatal aspect is made with dentin material and only the buccal surface is veneered with enamel material.

Performing the layering technique skillfully requires quite a bit of hands-on experience once the principle is understood. A good exercise to learn about the optical characteristics of the composite is to make composite teeth. To do this, a silicone impression is made from the palatal aspect of an extracted incisor, and then the root is made out of an

Fig 2-9 Exercise to learn the layering technique: Build a tooth with composite. This composite tooth was made with Artemis (Ivoclar Vivadent).

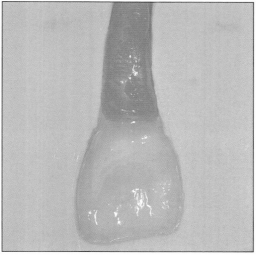

Fig 2-9a Silicone form in which the root was created with a dark, opaque composite. The palatal and proximal enamel are reconstructed with a thin layer of enamel composite (13% to 15% translucency).

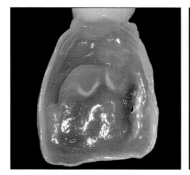 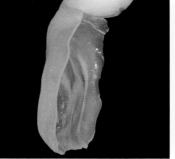 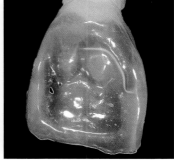

Fig 2-9b After light curing, the silicone form may be removed. Note how thin the enamel shell is (view from buccal aspect).

Fig 2-9c The side view clearly shows how the proximal shape is formed with a thin layer of enamel composite.

Fig 2-9d View from the palatal aspect.

opaque, rather dark composite material (Fig 2-9a). To start forming the crown, the palatal and proximal enamel composite (13% to 15% translucency) is placed against the silicone model (Figs 2-9b to 2-9d). The dentin core is built up with different layers of dentin composite (7% to 8% translucency) (Figs 2-9e to 2-9h).

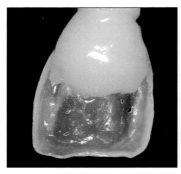

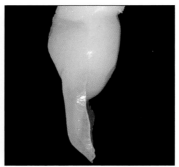

Fig 2-9e The cervical part of the core of the tooth is applied with a dentin composite (7% to 8% translucency).

Fig 2-9f The correct thickness of the tooth is checked in the side view.

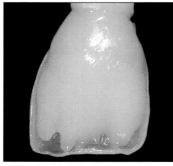

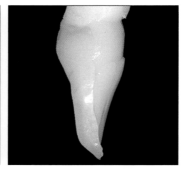

Fig 2-9g The cervical portion of the dentin core is built up with a slightly lighter dentin composite. Note the modeling of the mamelons.

Fig 2-9h The correct profile is checked in the side view.

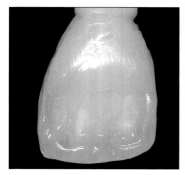

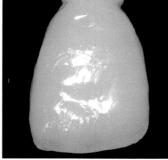

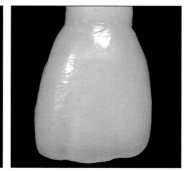

Fig 2-9i Now the incisal edge is constructed with clear composite (30% translucency).

Fig 2-9j The complete buccal surface is now covered with enamel composite (13% to 15% translucency).

Fig 2-9k Finished composite crown after structuring the surface (macro- and microstructure) and final polishing.

Fig 2-10 Reconstruction of the incisal edge of a maxillary right central incisor. The old restoration is unsatisfactory in both function and esthetics. This restoration was made with Mirus (Coltène, Altstätten, Switzerland).

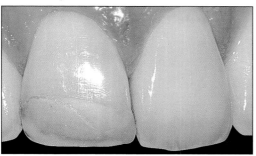

Fig 2-10a The first step is to determine the color. Instead of using only a shade guide, a composite mockup made with all layers in the desired colors can aid in confirming color selection.

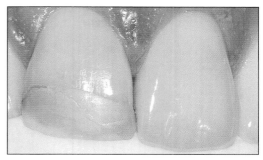

Fig 2-10b A silicone stent, made with a putty silicone impression material, will aid in determining the correct position of the incisal edge.

"Clear" composite may be used for the incisal edge, especially to create a tooth for a young individual (Fig 2-9i). The last layer is made with enamel composite (Fig 2-9j). After characterization of the surface with macrostructures (indentations) and microstructures (scratches and pits) and final polishing with the Occlubrush (Kerr), the composite tooth looks very natural (Fig 2-9k).

A clinical case in which an insufficient restoration was replaced demonstrates the three-layer technique (Fig 2-10). The most important first step is to determine the tooth color (Fig 2-10a). This can be done with a shade guide. However, the best way is to make a mockup by quickly placing a restoration with the intended layers, applied in one operation (all layers on top of each other), and then curing it. Since no adhesive is used, the mockup can be easily removed by shearing it off with a scaler.

In the present case, a dentin A3 and three different enamel shades are selected. A silicone stent made with a putty silicone impression material is then prepared (Fig 2-10b). This serves as a form to produce the palatal contour of the restoration. This is important, because it guarantees the correct position of the incisal edge. Nothing is more disturbing than creating a pleasing reconstruction and then being forced, due to functional requirements, to grind it thin on the palatal side or short on the incisal edge. If the shape of the old restoration is inappropriate, it must be corrected beforehand. This can be done with the mockup (only the palatal form must be correct) or with boxing wax (Kerr).

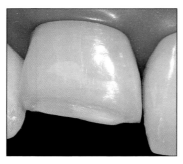

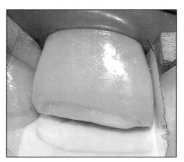

Fig 2-10c Cavity preparation. Only short bevels are prepared.

Fig 2-10d Incisions in the silicone stent allow perfect placement of matrix bands. Wooden wedges should be shortened so that the silicone stent is not displaced. With this technique an ideal form for placing the initial palatal layer of enamel composite is created.

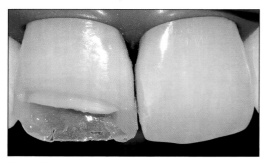

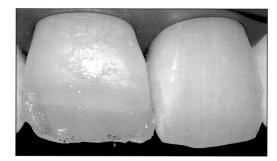

Fig 2-10e The palatal and proximal enamel shell is placed. Two different enamel shades are used.

Fig 2-10f The first dentin layer is placed.

After the cavity is prepared with short bevels (Fig 2-10c), the silicone stent is placed, and with incisions in the silicone, the matrix bands can be perfectly placed to produce the palatal and proximal contours of the reconstruction (Fig 2-10d). The palatal and proximal enamel shell is then made by placing enamel composite against this form (Fig 2-10e). The dentin core is then placed in different layers, if needed (Fig 2-10f), and some characterization may be added with intensive stain (Fig 2-10g). Finally, the buccal surface is layered with enamel composite (Fig 2-10h), and after the last layer is cured, the restoration is completed with surface characterization and final polishing (Fig 2-10i).

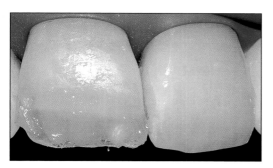

Fig 2-10g Some characterization is made with intensive stain. Note that these intensive colors must be used with discretion. They are best applied with a thin artist's paintbrush.

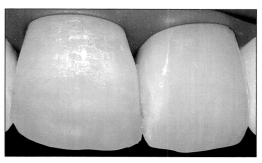

Fig 2-10h The buccal surface is finalized with two different enamel shades.

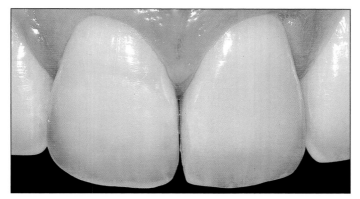

Fig 2-10i Completed restoration after final polishing.

If teeth are not very transparent, or if there is insufficient space, excellent results can be obtained with a two-layer technique. A similar clinical case demonstrates the possibilities of this approach (Fig 2-11). In contrast to the three-layer technique, in this technique the entire palatal aspect of the restoration is built up with dentin composite. The desired transparency of the incisal edge determines whether the dentin material is applied flush with the incisal edge or stopped short of it. The remainder of the restoration is then built up with enamel composite only.

Fig 2-11 Reconstruction of an incisal edge with a two-layer technique. This restoration was made with Artemis.

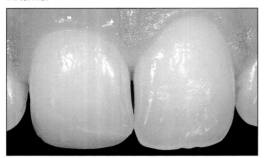

Fig 2-11a This restoration no longer fulfilled the patient's esthetic expectations.

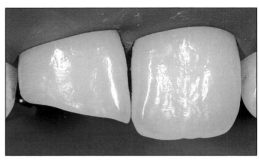

Fig 2-11b Cavity preparation.

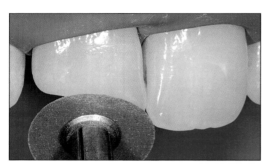

Fig 2-11c A short bevel is prepared with an aluminum oxide–coated disk.

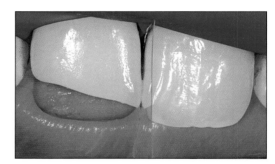

Fig 2-11d A silicone stent is prepared to determine the incisal edge.

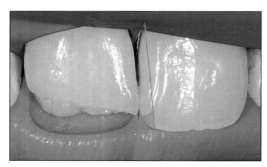

Fig 2-11e The dentin core is built up against the silicone stent using dentin composite (7% to 8% translucency).

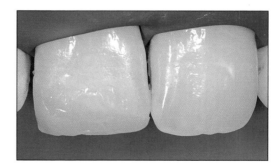

Fig 2-11f The entire incisal edge is built up with enamel composite (13% to 15% translucency).

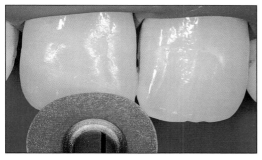

Fig 2-11g The final contouring of the buccal surface is best performed with an aluminum oxide–coated disk.

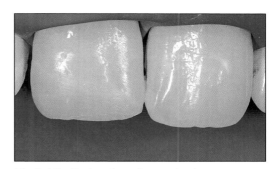

Fig 2-11h Restoration after contouring.

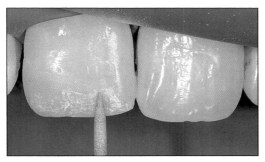

Fig 2-11i Surface structure is created with a fine-grain diamond bur.

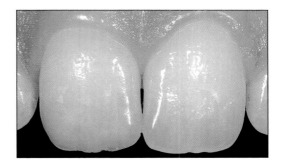

Fig 2-11j The finished restoration is well-integrated in function and esthetics.

Conclusions

Using small-particle hybrid composites with the appropriate handling technology, clinicians are able to produce invisible restorations. The layering technique, which uses not only different colors but also, most importantly, different translucencies of the composites, is a key for success. These techniques are demanding and time-consuming, and therefore the cost for the patient is high.

References

1. Rufenacht CL. Fundamentals of Esthetics. Chicago: Quintessence, 1990.

2. Rufenacht CL. Principles of Esthetic Integration. Chicago: Quintessence, 2000.

3. Buonocore MG. A simple method of increasing the adhesion of acrylic filling materials to enamel surfaces. J Dent Res 1955;34:849–853.

4. Nakabayashi N, Kojima K, Masuhara E. The promotion of adhesion by the infiltration of monomers into tooth substrates. J Biomed Mater Res 1982;16:265–273.

5. Van Meerbeek B, Inokoshi SM, Braem M, Lambrechts P, Vanherle G. Morphological aspects of the resin-dentin interdiffusion zone with different dentin adhesive systems. J Dent Res 1992; 71:1530–1540.

6. Van Meerbeek B, Dhem A, Goret-Nicaise M, Braem M, Lambrechts P, Vanherle G. Comparative SEM and TEM examination of the ultrastructure of the resin-dentin interdiffusion zone. J Dent Res 1993;72:495–501.

7. Roulet J-F. Degradation of dental polymers. Basel, Switzerland: Karger, 1987.

8. Davidson CL, De Gee AJ, Feilzer A. The competition between the composite dentin bond strength and polymerization contraction stress. J Dent Res 1984;63:1396–1399.

9. Yoshikawa T, Burrow MF, Tagami J. The effects of bonding system and light curing method on reducing stress of different c-factor cavities. J Adhes Dent 2001;3:177–184.

10. Davidson CL, De Gee AJ. Light-curing units, polymerization, and clinical implications. J Adhes Dent 2000;2:167–174.

11. Gagliani M, Fadini L, Ritzmann JM. Depth of cure efficacy of high-power curing devices vs traditional halogen lamps. J Adhes Dent 2002; 4:41–48.

12. Van Meerbeek B, Yoshida Y, Snauwaert J, et al. Hybridization effectiveness of a two-step versus a three-step smear layer removing adhesive system examined correlatively by TEM and AFM. J Adhes Dent 1999;1:7–23.

13. Brännström M, Linden LA, Aström A. The hydrodynamics of the dental tubule and of pulp fluid. Caries Res 1967;1:310–317.

14. Brännström M. Communication between the oral cavity and the dental pulp associated with restorative treatment. Oper Dent 1984;9:57–68.

15. Bergmann P, Noack MJ, Roulet J-F. Marginal adaptation with glass-ceramic inlays adhesively luted with glycerine gel. Quintessence Int 1991; 22:739–744.

16. Feilzer AJ, De Gee AJ, Davidson CL. Setting stress in composite resin in relation to configuration of the restoratives. J Dent Res 1987;66: 1636–1639.

17. Dietschi D, Spreafico R. Adhesive Metal-Free Restorations. Chicago: Quintessence, 1994.

Chapter 3

Preservation of Enamel with Precise Tooth Preparation

Galip Gürel

Abstract

To achieve outstanding esthetic qualities, porcelain laminate veneers require minimum tooth reduction. Even though the technique for these restorations may seem easy, it requires very delicate and precise tooth preparation. Depending on the difficulty of the case, a space of 0.3 to 0.9 mm must be provided so that the dental technician can perform the layering technique. Different tools can be used to make exact preparation depths. This chapter describes a practical technique to achieve precise tooth preparation, thus minimizing unnecessary tooth reduction. The technique also gives the clinician the opportunity to visualize the final esthetic outcome even before the teeth are prepared.

Two important revolutions—implants and bonding—have completely changed the image of traditional dentistry. When we look back at dentistry 25 years ago and compare the differences with modern dentistry, the effects that these two methods have had are vividly apparent. This chapter is not about implants but about esthetic dentistry, a concept that grew tremendously after bonding was introduced.

Porcelain Laminate Veneers and Bonding

Esthetic dentistry owes a great deal to pioneers like Pincus, who in 1938 tried plastic veneers on Hollywood celebrities even before other clinicians were aware of bonding[1]; like Buonocore, who proved in 1955 that teeth can be etched and bonded[2]; like Rochette in 1975[3] and Calamia, Simonsen, and others, who proved that porcelain can be etched and then bonded to composites.[4,5] These revolutionary advances set the stage for other techniques, such as porcelain laminate veneers (PLVs), which are capable of restoring not only the esthetics of teeth but also their function.

These new techniques needed further advancement. In the early years of PLVs, bonding was mainly limited to the enamel surface, which limited the area of the indications. However, the introduction of the wet-bonding technique by Kanca[6] provided the opportunity to bond to dentin in high megapascals, which expanded the areas in which PLVs or bonded porcelain restorations[7] can be utilized today. Resin composite, acid-etched porcelain, and etched enamel have been proven in in vitro studies to create a strong, durable complex.[8,9] In this process of ceramic restoration, the calcified dental tissue, the ceramic, and the bonding materials are the three main components, with the interface between the bonding agent and the ceramic being another factor. This well-structured ensemble is able to withstand the forces of mechanical stress (knock or mechanical fatigue), thermal stress (mechanical fatigue), or hydric stress (infiltration and sorption) existing in the oral environment.[10] By means of a micromechanic interlocking, a bond of 20 MPa was obtained between composite luting resins and purely inorganic enamel.[11,12] The bond strength to etched and silanated ceramics has been reported as high as 45 MPa.[13] These bond-strength values are high enough to resist "tensile and shear forces that are generated by thermal ex-

pansion or by shrinkage during the polymerization of composites."[14]

Bonded porcelain restorations, in addition to their outstanding esthetic qualities, need minimal invasive preparation,[15] especially compared with complete-crown restorations. This is their greatest advantage.

In fact, in the early 1980s some authors[16–18] recommended no tooth preparation at all for PLV applications. However, such applications result in a bulky PLV surface that appears too large in the mouth; the excessive emergence profile creates contours that might distort the gingival tissues.

In time the technique changed a bit, and many authors[19–25] agreed that the tooth surface should be prepared to a certain extent, but in the least invasive way possible. Various PLV preparation sets were introduced to the dental market, and almost all of them had depth cutters that limited clinicians' efforts to prepare the tooth surface more than necessary.

The average thickness of a PLV, depending on the material to be used, varies from 0.3 to 0.9 mm. This is why depth cutters are used. Once the desired depth is approached, the rest of the preparation is completed with a round-ended fissure diamond bur, which will reduce the excess enamel to a level indicated by the depth cutter. The use of standardized objects to allow size or angle judgment by direct comparison improves accuracy, and their routine use may improve the quality of the restorative treatment. Two different-sized depth cutters (no. 868A.314.018 and no. 868A.314.021, Komet, Lemgo, Germany) control the depth of the facial tooth preparation. They enable the clinician to quantify enamel reduction, guide, and visualize. With use of the rounded tip, margins can be plotted if necessary. When the color changes are two shades or less,[23] as in more than 90% of cases, 0.3- and 0.5-mm depth cutters are used. Without a depth guide, it can be detrimental to gauge reduction in enamel depth between 0.3 and 0.5 mm.[26] However, if the preoperative evaluation is not done properly, these depth cutters can destroy sound tooth structure and thus weaken the intact tooth structure. That would be a great method if all the teeth to be veneered were aligned perfectly on the dental arch and had no facial enamel loss (eg, due to aging).

Preventive dentistry enables patients to retain their natural teeth until much more advanced ages. Nowadays, teeth are being restored with fixed prosthodontics instead of removable dentures.

However, during the body's natural aging process, tooth structure also ages. The physiologic aging of teeth is indicated by a darkening of the tooth (high in chroma), as a result of the volumetric enamel loss of the facial surface of the tooth. Thus, the thinner the enamel, the darker the dentin shows through. After years of grinding and bruxing, the incisal edges tend to become shorter and shorter, giving an aged look to the mouth when the lips are relaxed and the teeth are not visible. Additional enamel loss especially is underestimated when a tooth is being prepared for PLVs. When the teeth are prepared without consideration to the already reduced enamel structure, the preparation will most probably end on the dentin surface and unnecessary sound tooth structure will be lost; in other words, the preparation of the teeth will be excessive.

Enamel-Dentin Structure

As we know, enamel and dentin are two different substrates. Enamel has a hard structure and can resist occlusal forces, but it is fragile and can crack easily. On the other hand, dentin is flexible but is not wear-resistant without the enamel structure to protect it. Together they form a "composite" structure, which is the unique characteristic of the tooth.[27]

As Lin and his colleagues have explained, the junction of the enamel and dentin (DEJ) has a very effective and interesting form, referred to as the *fibril-reinforced bond*.[28] This special bonding prevents the progression of enamel cracks to the dentin structure. The DEJ serves as a barrier. In other words, the DEJ plays a significant role in assisting stress transfer and in resisting enamel crack propagation.[29] This means that clinicians must avoid preparation on the DEJ by keeping the preparation lines in enamel as much as possible.

The flexibility of dentin, combined with the rigidity and strength of enamel, creates a balance in the crown's flexibility. As the enamel surface is reduced during the aging process, the flexibility of the tooth increases. Magne et al used both strain-gauge experiments and finite element models to demonstrate the significant effect of the enamel shell on stress distribution.[7,30] If there has been a volumetric loss of the enamel shell, the original enamel structure and rigidity balance of the crown must be restored.

Enamel is vital for the protection of the tooth. Iatrogenic factors must be prevented to maintain as much of the enamel structure as possible. When the tooth is restored with the proper porcelain materials that possess the same strength as the enamel, the original tooth fiber–reinforcement can be achieved again.[31,32] These parameters illustrate the importance of precise preparations for PLV restorations. To prevent excess tooth reduction, and to maintain the DEJ and most of the original tooth structure, clinicians must make meticulous treatment plans.

Tooth Preparation for Porcelain Laminate Veneers

To maximize esthetics, improve fracture resistance, optimize laboratory artistry, and maintain soft tissue health, meticulous tooth preparation is required for PLVs.[33] Although PLVs can be applied with very little tooth preparation, this procedure should not be misinterpreted as simple; in fact it requires great skill, control, and training because no corrections can be made once the procedure is completed.[26] Experience is required to master 0.3- to 0.5-mm reductions. However, with some special techniques, which will be explained later, even inexperienced clinicians can achieve predictable preparations. Various kinds of PLV preparation and finishing kits are available to help the dentist achieve success through systematic procedures.

Tooth Position

The position and alignment of teeth in the arch can significantly affect the appearance and balance of a smile. A rotated or lingually or facially positioned or

aligned tooth will disrupt the total harmony and balance. A smile is more pleasant when the teeth are adequately positioned and aligned. Poorly positioned or rotated teeth not only distort the shape of the arch, but they also interfere with their apparent relative proportion. Anterior esthetics necessitates the contouring and shaping of the teeth to create the illusion of pretty teeth and an attractive smile.

One of the crucial issues in the production of PLVs is to maintain the maximum amount of existing enamel. Before the clinician even begins treatment planning, especially when treating the aged tooth, the amount of remaining enamel and the final volume of the PLV should be carefully analyzed. Tooth preparation that is done without prior evaluation and planning will have a negative effect on the final result.[34]

The amount of necessary tooth reduction should be determined not by the existing tooth surface but rather by the final volume of the restoration. The spatial orientation and architectural dimensions of the waxup will be used to predesign and validate the intended preparations for the teeth involved. This illustrates the importance of using the correct waxup techniques to create the exact tooth shape desired. In porcelain veneer treatment, the most important element in the process is the waxup.[35]

Closing Diastemata

A common feature in the anterior dentition is the presence of diastemata. They distort a pleasing smile by interrupting the observer's view of the overall dental

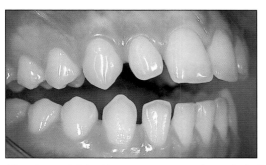 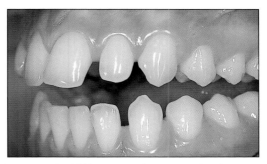

Figs 3-1 and 3-2 Diastema cases are the main indication group for PLVs; some others are color changes and malformed and misaligned teeth. Prior to beginning treatment of diastema cases, the proportion of the teeth should be carefully analyzed and a three-dimensional composite mockup must be made.

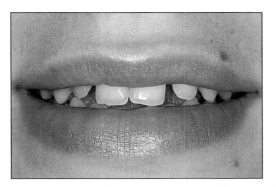 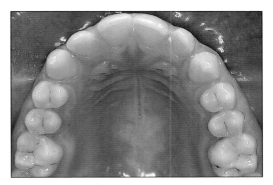

Figs 3-3 and 3-4 Diastemata are generally present between the central incisors because of the incisally attached frenulum. However, diastemata sometimes occur between the lateral incisors and canines. In such situations, the first step is usually orthodontic treatment, but in some social indications, as in this case of a fashion model, restoration of the anterior teeth with PLVs is a far better solution.

composition (Figs 3-1 and 3-2). Closing a diastema is one of the most common indications for PLVs.

Diastemata generally occur when the frenulum is positioned incisally between the central incisors. However, in some cases, the diastema occurs instead between the lateral and central incisors or the lateral incisor and the canine (Figs 3-3 and 3-4). This type of case needs meticu-

lous preparation and effective communication with the laboratory to achieve the desired result and to avoid unpleasant situations for the clinician and patient. Whether the case is simple or complicated, careful planning, effective communication, and unified decision making by the patient, technician, and clinician are vital prior to the commencement of the treatment.

The space created by the diastema should be closed proportionally and distributed among the anterior teeth. Trying to close the entire gap with one or two veneers is a common mistake made by some clinicians and will result in an overcompensation of the original problem.[36] Sometimes restoration may involve more than one or two teeth on either side of the diastema.

The width of the teeth is affected by their apparent size. Teeth with identical widths but different lengths will appear to have different widths.[37] This is an important principle to remember when closing diastemata in the anterior region, because an alteration will be introduced in the length-width relationship and can unfavorably alter the smile.[38]

During the first appointment with the patient, instant-developing and digital photographs of the patient's mouth and face must be taken from various angles. These visual aids are necessary because study casts alone are not sufficient for the technician to create esthetic results. For this reason, the laboratory must be fully informed with the necessary tools.

Composite Mockup

After photographs have been taken, the first step is to prepare a composite mockup in the patient's mouth. The mockup enables the patient and the clinician to roughly evaluate the effect the new restoration will have on the patient's appearance, function, and phonetic pronunciation.[39] In other words, the composite mockup is a valuable aid; it gives an immediate idea of what the eventual outcome will be.[40] The mockup may not al-

ways be satisfying to the patient. During the mockup stage, no tooth reduction is performed; therefore, if there are any protrusive teeth in the arch, the mockup will not give a clear picture of the final result.

However, the mockup will provide a rough idea of what can be expected and prepare both the patient and the clinician for the changes that are about to occur. Both parties will then be better able to decide whether to continue with the planned treatment. From the preparation to the PLV buildup to finishing of the restoration, the clinician is guided by these spatial references. The restorative steps will be facilitated by the visual inspection of the frontal, lateral, and incisal planes.[41]

Short-Term Provisionals

When the teeth need to be lengthened and/or protruded, some patients may complain that the pressure on the upper lip causes phonetic disturbances.[42] In such cases, the mockups can be held in place for a longer period of time. Light retention can be provided by extending the composite over the space where the interdental contact area ends apically and the papillae begin, or by other undercuts incorporated into the composite buildup. The patient may then wear the mockups for up to a few hours to better evaluate the esthetic outcome. During this time, the patient can become accustomed to the uncomfortable pressure of the mockups on the lips, as well as get feedback from people they trust about the proposed esthetic outcome. This is all done for the benefit of the patient, out of respect for his or her desire for a functional

Fig 3-5 The impression of patient's maxillary and mandibular teeth is identical to the composite mockups that are transferred to the laboratory. The technician must prepare the waxup on the casts made from these impressions. While preparing the waxup, the technician is free to cut back the protrusive teeth on the model. After putting the protrusive teeth into their proper position, the technician prepares the waxup according to the composite mockup the clinician provided. The technician must prepare a silicone index that wraps this waxup. The dentist can also prepare the silicone index chairside, in minutes, with putty silicone.

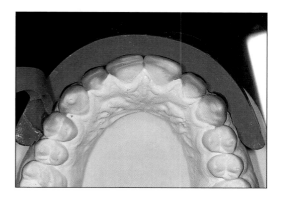

esthetic goal.[43] The clinician should use the mockup, if for no other reason, for the educational and enlightening experience it offers the patient.[44]

Waxup

The second step is to take an impression of the teeth, with and without the mockup in place. With the aid of instant-developing and digital photographs, the information can be sent to the laboratory in a matter of seconds, enabling the clinician and technician to discuss and decide on the waxup. The composite mockup will act as the reference that enables the technician to correct the protrusive and labial positions, and more important, the position of the incisal edge.

In cases that involve protruding teeth, following the communication about the case, the technician may cut the protrusive teeth on the model according to the

dental arch that has been planned. The reduction must also be made according to the space necessary for the PLV. The technician then makes the necessary reduction of enamel on all remaining teeth on the model, prepares a waxup on that model, and sends the waxup model to the clinic.[35]

Silicone Index and Transparent Template

For precise evaluation, in addition to the waxup, transparent templates and the silicone index are necessary. These two diagnostic aids are prepared from the waxup and sent to the clinic (Fig 3-5).[45] The transparent template will be used in the fabrication of the provisional restorations. The silicone index will be essential in determining whether the preparations have been successfully completed.

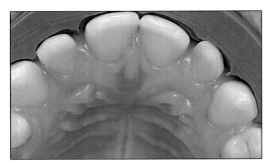

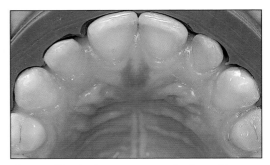

Fig 3-6 When this silicone index is placed on the teeth, the primary contacts between the protrusive teeth and the index can be observed. Here, the primary contact of the mesial surface of the left lateral incisor is evident.

Fig 3-7 "Aesthetic pre-recontouring" must be performed on the protrusive teeth. The points of the teeth that are in contact with the index are cut back until no primary contact exists. While doing this tooth reduction, each tooth, such as the maxillary right lateral incisor and the distal of the left central and right lateral incisors, must be verified with the "aesthetic pre-evaluative temporaries."

Aesthetic Pre-recontouring

The third step is tooth preparation. Even in the simplest case, there are numerous details to attend to. The first detail is to remove the necessary amount of protruding enamel according to the information provided by the waxup. Referred to as "aesthetic pre-recontouring" (APR), this step enables clinicians to esthetically correct the position of the protruded teeth on the dental arch.[46] The silicone index acts as the guide for the clinician during the removal of the enamel, especially in the case of the protrusive tooth. When the silicone index is placed over the unprepared teeth, the clinician can clearly see which teeth are the cause of an incorrect fit and which teeth will need additional reduction (Fig 3-6).

Until the correct fit of the silicone index is acquired, the teeth must be slowly and carefully reduced (Fig 3-7). Before the actual material preparation of teeth can begin, the transparent template is placed over the teeth and observed for a proper fit. If the teeth have not been properly prepared, it will be difficult (if not impossible) to fit the template over the teeth, since the protruded parts of the teeth will create retentive areas.

Aesthetic Pre-evaluative Temporaries

The facial surfaces of the teeth are spot etched to provide a rough surface for the bonding of the "aesthetic pre-evaluative temporary" (APT) (Fig 3-8). Bonding materials are applied to the rough surface of the teeth and light cured. The transparent template is filled with flowable composite, placed over the unprepared

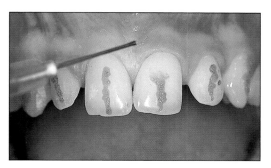

Fig 3-8 To lightly bond the APT before the teeth are prepared, the surfaces must be etched and adhesive applied.

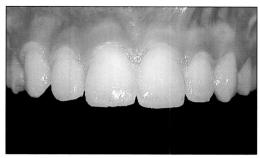

Fig 3-9 Application of the APT to the teeth. The proposed PLVs can be easily evaluated with the use of an APT. First, the clinician must check the incisal edge positions. At the same time, he can analyze whether the diastemata close in the correct proportion. Anterior guidance and the occlusion are roughly checked. The patient's phonetics and the harmony of the new smile with the patient's face are then evaluated.

teeth, and light cured.[46] Throughout the preparation, there is no need to anesthetize the patient. This is an advantage because the patient has full control over the lips and mouth, enabling the clinician and patient to freely observe the APT that was made from the transparent template.

The role of the APT is very important at this stage as it provides an opportunity for the clinician and patient to observe the approximate final result before the actual material preparation is made. The APT allows the clinician and patient to see the final result with the face, mouth, and tooth proportion, and to verify the incisal edge position. To determine whether the waxup is realistic in terms of occlusion, the patient is asked to perform protrusive and lateral excursions.

At this stage, the patient is given the opportunity to voice opinions or to re-

quest any changes. Although it is rare that the patient does not like the new smile (since it has been designed according to the initial composite mockup), changes can be made to the surface texture, forms, concavities, and the incisal length, so that the clinician and the patient are satisfied with the smile. If many changes are made to the APT, the new outcome of the teeth must be transferred to the laboratory, so that the ceramist is informed of the final decision (Fig 3-9).

Depth Cutter

To make minimally invasive preparations, PLV preparation sets were created by the pioneers in this field and are available. Although the sets may consist of different types of burs, most of them contain

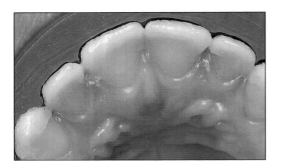

Fig 3-10 To determine if the APT is properly placed on the teeth, the silicone index must be seated over the APT. If both of them are seated properly, the silicone index must exhibit a passive fit with the APT.

the "depth cutter" bur, which enables tooth reduction at the proper depth. The shaft of these burs does not cut the tooth structure, while the rounded diamond coated rings help to cut down to the proper depth on the facial surface of the tooth.[26] Because depth cutters are different sizes, the clinician must decide which size to use to prevent excess reduction of the enamel or dentin and/or cause an excess porcelain thickness.

Following this, the entire facial surface is reduced to the grooves prepared by the depth cutter, using a round-ended fissure diamond bur. Of course, there are some disadvantages to depth cutters. The depth cutters are effective and useful if all the teeth are aligned properly on the maxillary or mandibular arch and no changes to form and position are necessary. However, when working on more complicated cases, such as aged or rotated teeth, careless use of the depth cutters may cause permanent damage to the teeth, resulting in unnecessary reduction of healthy tooth structure. The most predictable solution is to make the reductions with the aid of APTs.

Preparation with APTs

The major advantage of using the APT is to ensure that the final outcome is accepted by both the clinician and the patient. Since the APT now mimics the final contours of the actual PLVs, the teeth can be prepared precisely with the use of the APT.[46] To confirm whether the transparent template was applied in the mouth properly, the exact facial thickness achieved, and the APR and APT made properly, the silicone index must be placed over the APTs and its precise fit checked (Fig 3-10). The APT's facial thickness and the use of depth cutters will dictate the necessary facial reduction. In doing so the clinician will avoid the unnecessary loss of enamel associated with excessive tooth preparation and be able to supply the ideal preparation depth and volume for PLV production. One should never forget that the most important factor concerning the nature of the PLV is that it cannot be thinned down or shortened without seriously affecting the outer surface, incisal edge, or general esthetics of the restoration.[26]

Fig 3-11 It is of the utmost importance that the teeth are prepared over the APT. Excess tooth reduction can be prevented by following this practice. The first reduction is done with depth cutters, as if preparing the original tooth structure. Since the APT mimics the convexity of the original tooth, the depth cutter must be applied in the different angles on the incisal, facial, and gingival thirds.

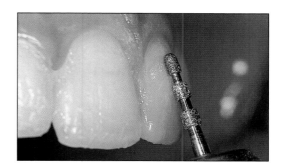

It is recommended that the silicone index be used to check tooth reduction systematically.[47] This systematic check enables the clinician to reduce the proper amount of tooth structure on all teeth. However, there is one disadvantage to this method: As it is the clinician who checks the silicone index after the reduction, those who are inexperienced in PLV procedures may be unaware that they have made excessive tooth reductions between steps, possibly resulting in permanent damage to the teeth.

Even simple mistakes can be prevented by the use of an APT. According to the author's experience, this method provides predictable tooth preparation that perfectly fits the newly designed restorations.[46] The most important feature of this method is that the teeth can be prepared over the APTs, which are nearly identical to the final porcelain restorations. This prevents excessive tooth reduction, especially for the lingually positioned teeth. The author believes that tooth preparation with APTs is the most important stage and that it provides the most precise and predictable minimally invasive tooth reductions.

The clinician now instinctively focuses on the preparation of the facial side of the tooth according to the final volumetric outcome. Especially in the case of rotated teeth, the facial aspects, which are positioned lingually on the dental arch, need little or no reduction. Tooth reduction with the help of the depth cutters over the APT enables the clinician to achieve an accurate, minimally invasive preparation for the final restoration.

Facial Preparation

Depth cutters are used as if preparing the real tooth structure (Fig 3-11). The APT mimics the facial contours of the final restorations and has the necessary convexity. The depth cutter bur must be used at different angles to create grooves of the same depth and following the facial convexity that the APT dictates. After the grooves have been prepared with the depth cutters, the entire facial surface can be painted for better visualization. In some cases it may be surprising to see that lingually positioned portions of some teeth have not been reached with the depth cutter (Fig 3-12). These

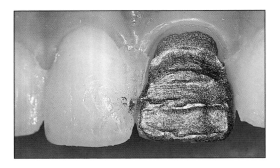

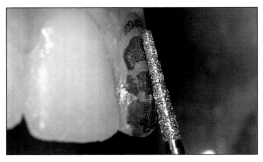

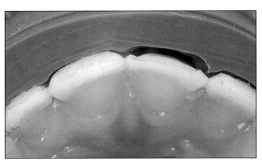

Fig 3-12 To visualize the reduction of the tooth structure done with the depth cutter, the tooth surface can be painted with gold paint. If the tooth is dramatically rotated or palatally positioned, further reduction can be done only on the APT, not on the tooth itself.

Fig 3-13 With a round-ended bur, the facial surface must be prepared until no paint remains. At this level, it is certain that the proper reduction of the tooth, referred to as the actual material preparation, can be made. Now the clinician has achieved minimal tooth reduction, and there is enough space for the technician to prepare the PLV.

Fig 3-14 After the facial surface preparation, the clinician must check the preparation with the silicone index seated on the remaining APT. Generally, it is evident that equal space has been prepared between the prepared surfaces of the APT and the silicone index in order to obtain a PLV of uniform thickness.

areas really do not need to be prepared. However, to ensure the bond strength of the resin composite to the tooth surface, it is necessary to reduce the enamel.[9,48,49] Because of its poor retention capacity, the aprismatic top surface of mature teeth that have not been prepared must be removed. Careful attention is of the utmost importance to obtain successful results and secure bonding.[50] Using the round-ended bur at different angles following the convexity, the APT must be cut back until no painted surface remains (Fig 3-13). When all the paint on the surface has been abraded, this is the essential depth determined with the guidance of the APT and the depth cutter. Depending on the choice of porcelain material and the amount of color change necessary, the essential depth can be anywhere from 0.3 to 0.9 mm.[26] After the facial surface has been prepared, the silicone index must be applied over the teeth to verify if the reduction is sufficient (Fig 3-14).

Incisal Edge Preparation

During preparation of the teeth over the APT, the detail that causes the most uncertainty is the incisal edge. Different types of incisal edge preparation have been developed, improved, and discussed by many renowned authors. Whether or not the incisal edge of the tooth should be included in the preparation of the PLV is still a matter of debate. Several authors favor the overlapped incisal preparation.[22,23,51] Some authors believe[52–54] that full coverage is vitally important to improve the mechanical resistance of the veneer, despite the fact that to accomplish this, 0.5 to 2.0 mm of intact incisal edge may have to be removed, placing the vulnerable cavosurface margin in an area of opposing tooth contact. It is better to incorporate an incisal overlap in the preparation, as the porcelain is stronger and produces a positive seat during the cementation process. The proper seating of the veneer is made possible by the vertical stop that the slight incisal overlap provides.[16] It is also emphasized that the incisal edge should be incorporated into the preparation only when occlusal or esthetic requirements mandate it.[55–58]

As far as the esthetic outcome and stability of the restoration, this author prefers the butt joint preparation technique. Because of the greater stress at the incisal edge of the veneer, clinical cohesive ceramic fractures can occur.[59] Instead of a chamfer margin that may weaken the final restoration, a flat shoulder should be used at the incisal edge.[60] Photoelastic studies have shown that a wide vertical stop prepared to resist loads by covering of the incisal edge lessens the stress concentration in them.[52] When this technique is combined with the preparation through the APT, the minimal invasiveness of the incisal edge preparation will pleasantly surprise the clinician.

To ensure that there is enough space for the technician to create the dentin, translucent, and transparent effects of the porcelain used in the layering technique on the incisal third, a butt joint must be prepared 2 mm short of the planned incisal edge position. When the APT technique is not used, most clinicians generally do this preparation without taking the original length of the tooth into consideration. For example, when the tooth's incisal edge is to be lengthened by only 2 mm, yet a 2-mm preparation is made, then 4 mm of unnecessary, wasted space are now present. By using the APT, the clinician can see just how little tooth reduction is actually needed. If the existing tooth length is 1.5 mm shorter than the expected outcome, then to achieve a 2-mm incisal reduction, only 0.5 mm of preparation is required (Fig 3-15).

During preparation of the incisal edge, work on the APT is done with a 4-mm-diameter diamond fissure bur, to the depth of its radius. The entire incisal edge can be cut back 2 mm while the APT is covering the tooth (Fig 3-16). The preparation can be done over the APT one tooth at a time, or the entire facial surface of the teeth and incisal edges can be prepared at once. When the APT is removed after preparation, the clinician will realize just how little has been cut at the incisal edge (Fig 3-17).

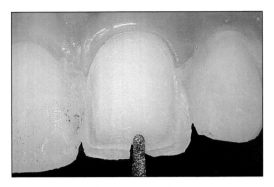

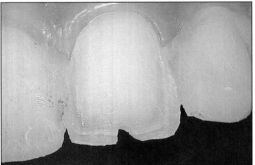

Fig 3-16 The APT on the left central and lateral incisors is reduced by 2 mm as if preparing the natural teeth.

Fig 3-15 Another effective way of using the APT is in the preparation of the incisal edges. About 2 mm of tooth reduction and a butt-joint preparation is necessary so that the technician can create the dentin effect on the PLVs. This is most precise if the APT is used.

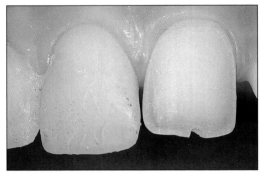

Fig 3-17 The APT is removed to show how little the natural tooth is reduced. This technique enables minimum tooth reduction and maximum space to be achieved.

Gingival Preparation

After the facial and incisal surface preparations have been completed, the APT must be removed to prepare the gingival third and the interproximal areas and to finalize the incisal surface of each tooth. To transfer a smooth gingival surface to the laboratory, the gingival third must be prepared with a fine, round-ended fissure diamond bur. Gingival contours should then be prepared 0.1 to 0.2 mm supragingivally if a dramatic color change is not needed (as in the case described in this chapter). This helps to prevent any possible periodontal problems and provides space for the thick emergence profiles. Although the preparation line is supragingival, it is almost impossible to detect the junction of the porcelain and the tooth after the PLV is bonded.

In the case of slight color changes, the preparation should be made level with the tip of the gingival sulcus as discussed above. However, in the case of a diastema, if the shape of the interdental papilla is not a clear triangle but is blunt, then the preparation must be made subgingivally (Fig 3-18). If some intentional pressure on the soft tissue is not made

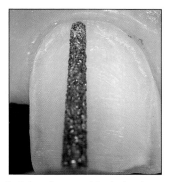

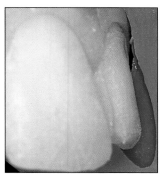

Fig 3-18 After the facial surface and incisal edges are prepared, the gingival and interproximal preparations are made. Even though preparation of the gingival area is done supragingivally at the area of closing, the gingival thirds that face the diastema are prepared subgingivally. The technician creates an overcontoured emergence profile on the porcelain restoration, and with light pressure the porcelain creates a triangular papilla.

Fig 3-19 The facial convexity and the amount of tooth reduction at the incisal edge are checked.

with the new restorations, the esthetic result will not be satisfactory, especially for the papilla, which will act like a squeezed balloon. In other words, if the preparation is limited to the facial, it will be physically impossible to apply pressure over the blunt gingiva and achieve the triangular form.[61]

Therefore, a small amount of subgingival preparation interproximally will enable the clinician to place the porcelain under the gingival tissue; this, in addition to the overcontouring the technician purposely left and the adjacent tooth, will push the papilla incisally and give the papilla a clear triangular shape. Hence, the subgingival preparation should not be limited to the imaginary interproximal contact area, but should also be extended toward the palate to create the intentional overcontouring of

the PLV between the buccal and palatal papilla.

For 100% predictability the distance between the interproximal intercrestal bone and the tip of the planned papilla should be 5 mm at most.[62] Otherwise, the papilla reshaped with this method may retract, forming black triangles. This distance must be determined before preparation, and accordingly the technician should decide where to make the interproximal contact points apically. These contact points should be at most 5 or 6 mm from the interproximal intercrestal bone.

After following these details and preparing the teeth, the clinician should check the preparation with the silicone index from various angles (Fig 3-19). From the profile view, the convexity of the facial surface must be parallel to the

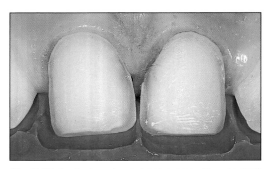

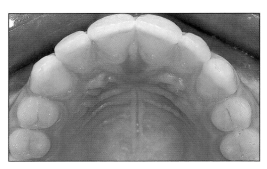

Fig 3-20 Incisal and proximal preparation control with the silicone index seated on the palatal surfaces of the teeth.

Fig 3-21 The occlusal alignment of the prepared teeth is confirmed.

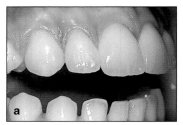
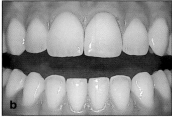
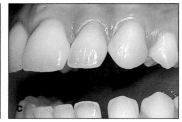

Figs 3-22a to 3-22c The final restoration has been achieved through diligent communication between the clinician, patient, and technician. When the proper amount of tooth structure is reduced, the technician can create a natural-looking PLV with the correct illusions and textures (technician: Gerard Ubassy). With such a meticulously planned treatment, the patient is satisfied with her new smile, and the dentist is pleased because the treatment was ethically planned using minimally invasive techniques while creating a beautiful smile.

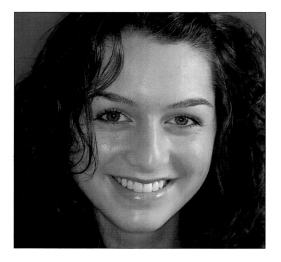

Fig 3-23 The harmony of the restorations with the patient's smile and face can be clearly seen.

silicone index. The incisal edges must be 2 mm shorter than the silicone index (Fig 3-20). At this point, the line of the butt joint between the facial surface and incisal edge must not be sharply angled. Otherwise, after the PLV is bonded, a horizontal line shadow will be visible under the laminate.

After the preparation and with the guide of the APT and the final check with the silicone index, the clinician undoubtedly will make the most minimally invasive and accurate preparation needed for the ceramist to make the PLVs with the layering technique. The rest depends on the technician's dedication, skills, knowledge, and desire to improve technical abilities. With such an efficient preparation, it is difficult for the laboratory to make mistakes.

Figure 3-21 demonstrates how perfect the occlusal arch can be when the teeth are restored with PLVs. The illusive effects, different color effects, and different proportions created with the layering technique provide a natural look with diastema cases (Figs 3-22a to 3-22c). After all, one of the most important components of a new smile design is its integration with the facial composition (Fig 3-23). All this effort will not mean much to a patient unless he or she feels comfortable and happy with the smile.

Conclusion

Esthetic dentistry is the aspect of dentistry for which patients most willingly come to the clinic. The patient's desires must be evaluated ethically and the patient's need for esthetic dentistry must be objectively determined. When clinicians decide on the indication of this treatment, they must then practice minimally invasive techniques. The PLV treatment is the most natural and esthetic solution for patients and especially for diastema cases. Since each tooth is connected to a human body, the clinician must always strive to make a minimally invasive preparation. Tooth preparation with the aid of APTs, which are prepared from the patient's individual waxup, provides the most predictable and precise tooth preparation and minimizes mistakes. In addition, it has been the author's experience that when the porcelain system to be used is determined before the teeth are prepared, the tooth preparations are minimally invasive.

References

1. Pincus CR. Building mouth personality. J South Calif Dent Assoc 1938;14:125–129.

2. Buonocore MG. A simple method of increasing the adhesion of acrylic filling materials to enamel surfaces. J Dent Res 1955;34:849–853.

3. Rochette AL. A ceramic restoration bonded by etched enamel and resin for fractured incisors. J Prosthet Dent 1975;33:287–293.

4. Simonsen RJ, Calamia JR. Tensile bond strength of etched porcelain [abstract 1154]. J Dent Res 1983;62:297.

5. Calamia JR, Vaidynathan TK, Hirsch SM. Shear strength of etched porcelains [abstract 64]. J Dent Res 1985;64:296.

6. Kanca J. Resin bonding to wet substrate. Bonding to dentin. Quintessence Int 1992;23:39–41.

7. Magne P, Douglas W. Porcelain veneer: Dentin bonding optimization and biomimetic recovery at the crown. Int J Prosthodont 1999;12:111–121.

8. Dumfart H, Schaffer H. Clinical analysis of ceramic bonding systems regarding shear force measurement. Dtsch Zahnarztl Z 1989;44:867–869.

9. Stacey GD. A shear stress analysis of the bonding of porcelain veneers to enamel. J Prosthet Dent 1993;70:395–402.

43

10. Picard B, Jardel V, Tirlet G. Ceramic bonding: Reliability. In: Degrange M, Roulet JF (eds). Minimally Invasive Restorations with Bonding. Berlin: Quintessence, 1997:103–129.

11. Gwinnett AJ. Interactions of dental materials with enamel. Trans Am Acad Dent Mater 1990; 3:30–35.

12. Anusavice KJ (ed). Nonaqueous elastomeric impression materials. Phillips' Science of Dental Materials, ed 10. Philadelphia: Saunders, 1996: 139–176.

13. Kern M, Thompson VP. Tensile bond strength of new adhesive systems to InCeram ceramic [abstract 2124]. J Dent Res 1993;72:369.

14. Feilzer AJ, De Gee AJ, Davidson CL. Increased wall-to-wall curing contraction in thin bonded resin layers. J Dent Res 1989;68:48–50.

15. Magne P, Douglas W. Design optimization and evolution of bonded ceramics for the anterior dentition. A finite-element analysis. Quintessence Int 1999;30:661–671.

16. Calamia JR. Etched porcelain facial veneers: A new treatment modality based on scientific and clinical evidence. N Y J Dent 1983;53:255–259.

17. Horn HR. Porcelain laminate veneers bonded to etched enamel. Dent Clin North Am 1983;27: 671–684.

18. Christensen GJ. Veneering the teeth. State of the art. Dent Clin North Am 1985;29:373–391.

19. Calamia JR. Etched porcelain veneers: The current state of the art. Quintessence Int 1985;16: 5–12.

20. Garber DA, Goldstein RE, Feinman RA. Porcelain Laminate Veneers. Chicago: Quintessence, 1987.

21. McComb D. Porcelain veneer technique: A promising new method for restoring strength and esthetics to damaged or discolored teeth. Ont Dent 1988;65:25–32.

22. Weinberg LA. Tooth preparation for porcelain laminates. N Y State Dent J 1989;5:25–28.

23. Nixon RL. Porcelain veneers: An esthetic therapeutic alternative. In: Rufenacht CR (ed). Fundamentals of Esthetics. Chicago: Quintessence, 1990:329–368.

24. Garber DA. Porcelain laminate veneers: To prepare or not to prepare? Compend Contin Educ Dent 1991;12:178–182.

25. Friedman MJ. Augmenting restorative dentistry with porcelain veneers. J Am Dent Assoc 1991; 122:29–34.

26. Touati B, Miara P, Nathanson D. Esthetic Dentistry and Ceramic Restorations. Singapore: Martin Dunitz, 1999:161–214.

27. Kraus BS, Jordan RE, Abrams L. Histology of the teeth and their investing structures. In: Kraus BS, Abrams L, Jordan RE (eds). Dental Anatomy and Occlusion: A Study of the Masticatory System. Baltimore: Williams and Wilkins, 1969:135.

28. Lin CP, Douglas WH, Erlandsen SL. Scanning electron microscopy of type I collagen at the dentin-enamel junction of human teeth. J Histochem Cytochem 1993;41:381–388.

29. Magne P, Belser U. Bonded Porcelain Restorations in the Anterior Dentition: A Biomimetic Approach. Berlin: Quintessence, 2002:23–56.

30. Magne P, Versilius A, Douglas WH. Rationalization of incisor shape: Experimental-numerical analysis. J Prosthet Dent 1999;81:345–355.

31. Reeh ES, Douglas WH, Messer HH. Stiffness of endodontically treated teeth related to restoration technique. J Dent Res 1989;68:1540–1544.

32. Linn J, Messer HH. Effect of restorative procedures on the strength of endodontically treated molars. J Endod 1994;20:479–485.

33. Chalifoux PR. Porcelain veneers. Curr Opin Cosmet Dent 1994:58–66.

34. Vence BS. Sequential tooth preparation for aesthetic porcelain full-coverage crown restorations. Pract Periodontics Aesthet Dent 2000;12: 77–85.

35. Magne P. Perspectives in esthetic dentistry. Quintessence Dent Technol 2000;23:86–89.

36. Goldstein RE. Esthetics in Dentistry, ed 2. Hamilton, Ontario, Canada: BC Decker, 1998: 123–133.

37. Yamamoto M, Miyoshi Y, Shiego K. Fundamentals of esthetics: Contouring techniques for metal-ceramic restorations. Quintessence Dent Technol 1990/1991;14:10–82.

38. Baratieri LN, Monteiro SJ, Andrada MA, Viera LC, Cardoso AC, Ritter AV. Esthetics: Direct Adhesive Restoration on Fractured Anterior Teeth. Santiago, Chile: Quintessence, 1998:35–75.

39. Dietschi D. Free-hand composite resin restorations: A key to anterior aesthetics. Pract Periodontics Aesthet Dent 1995;7:15–25.

40. Miller M. Cosmetic mock-ups. Reality 2000;14: 3203–3207.

41. Roulet JF, Degrange M. Adhesion—The Silent Revolution in Dentistry. Berlin: Quintessence, 2000:235–254.

42. Chiche GJ, Pinault A. Esthetics of Anterior Fixed Prosthodontics. Chicago: Quintessence, 1994:115–143.

43. Magne P, Perroud R, Hodges JS, Belser UC. Clinical performance of novel-design porcelain veneers for the recovery of coronal volume and length. Int J Periodontics Restorative Dent 2000;20:441–459.

44. Bliss CH. A philosophy of patient education. Dent Clin North Am 1960;(July):290.

45. Roach RR, Muia PJ. An esthetic checklist. In: Preston JD (ed). Perspectives in Dental Ceramics. Proceedings of the Fourth International Symposium on Ceramics. Chicago: Quintessence, 1988:445.

46. Gürel G. The Science and Art of Porcelain Laminate Veneers. Berlin: Quintessence, 2003: 215–308.

47. Magne P, Douglas WH. Additive contour of porcelain veneers: A key element in enamel preservation, adhesion, and esthetics for aging dentition. J Adhes Dent 1999;1:81–92.

48. Schneider PM, Messer LB, Douglas WH. The effect of enamel surface reduction in vitro on the bonding of composite resin to permanent human enamel. J Dent Res 1981;60:895–900.

49. Black JB. Esthetic restoration of tetracycline-stained teeth. J Am Dent Assoc 1982;104: 846–851.

50. Troedson M, Derand T. Shear stresses in the adhesive layer under porcelain veneers. A finite element method study. Acta Odontol Scand 1998;56:257–262.

51. Christensen GJ. Have porcelain veneers arrived? J Am Dent Assoc 1991;122:81.

52. Highton R, Caputo AA, Matjas J. A photoelastic study of stresses on porcelain laminate preparations. J Prosthet Dent 1987;58:157–161.

53. Chpindel P, Cristou M. Tooth preparation and fabrication of porcelain veneers using a double-layer technique. Pract Periodontics Aesthet Dent 1994;6:19–28.

54. Meijering AC, Roeters FJ, Mulder J, Creugers NH. Recognition of veneer restorations by dentists and beautician students. J Oral Rehabil 1997;24:506–511.

55. Nordbo H, Rygh-Thoresen N, Henaug T. Clinical performance of porcelain laminate veneers without incisal overlapping: 3-year results. J Dent 1994;22:342–345.

56. Karlsson S, Landahl I, Stegersjö G, Milleding P. A clinical evaluation of ceramic laminate veneers. Int J Prosthodont 1992;5:447–451.

57. Garber D. Porcelain laminate veneers: Ten years later. Part I: Tooth preparation. J Esthet Dent 1993;5:57–62.

58. Crispin BJ. Full veneers. The functional and esthetic application of bonded ceramics. Compend Contin Educ Dent 1994;15:284,286–294.

59. Freedman MJ. A 15-year test of porcelain veneer failure—A clinician's observations. Compend Contin Educ Dent 1998;19:625–686.

60. Castelnuovo J, Tjan AH, Philips K, Nicholls JI, Kois JC. Fracture load and mode of failure of ceramic veneers with different preparations. J Prosthet Dent 2000;83:171–180.

61. Sanavi F, Weisgold AS, Rose LF. Biologic width and its relation to periodontal biotypes. J Esthet Dent 1998;10:157–163.

62. Tarnow D, Stahl SS, Magner A, Zamzok J. Human gingival attachment responses to gingival crown placement—Marginal remodeling. J Clin Periodontol 1986;13:563–569.

Chapter 4

Changes in Operative Dentistry—Beyond G. V. Black

Graham J. Mount

Abstract

One hundred years have passed since G. V. Black suggested a classification of cavity designs that was intended to cover all possibilities for the treatment of a carious lesion. Over the succeeding century there has been considerable progress in the understanding of the caries process: Fluoride can be incorporated as an integral part of caries control; there is a better understanding of the bacteriology of the caries process; and modification of the oral flora is possible. There has also been continuing change in the methods of cavity preparation, limited modification in cavity design, and the introduction of adhesive restorative materials. It would appear that the only items that have remained unchanged are the design and classification of cavities, and now is the time to modify the classification. It would seem more logical to classify the lesions in relation to the tooth surfaces on which they are likely to appear rather than continue to use a classification that was designed essentially for the placement of amalgam. It must be acknowledged that removal of tooth structure by surgical means cannot be regarded as a satisfactory method for control of a disease that is bacterial in origin. Conservation of natural tooth structure should be the first priority.

In the early 1880s Miller[1] and Black[2] first identified the bacterial strains associated with the development of dental caries and suggested that it was lactic acid produced by these bacteria that brought about the dissolution of dentin. Shortly thereafter Miller noted that lactic acid could also decalcify enamel, and he identified the places on the crown of a tooth that were most likely to suffer from acid attack. Over the next decade G. V. Black rationalized this knowledge into his theory of "extension for prevention" and developed a classification of cavity designs for the control of caries. At that time the restorative materials were limited to amalgam, gold, and silicate cement.

With that level of knowledge the proposed cavity designs were logical. The dimensions of the cavity, in both width and depth, were controlled by the need to place and condense amalgam or to construct a gold inlay. The use of dovetail designs and mechanical interlocks was dictated by the need for physical retention of materials that were not inherently adhesive. The suggestion of extension for prevention was a necessary corollary to the lack of understanding of the caries process.

Progress in these basic principles over the first half of the last century has been limited. The methods of using rotary cutting instruments improved from foot-activated machines so that, by the end of the 1920s, electrically driven machines were commonplace. The speed was limited by the rather unsophisticated cord-and-pulley drive system, and it was another 20 years before diamond[3] and tungsten carbide[4] cutting instruments became freely available. In the late 1940s methods for increasing the speed of cutting, necessitating water cooling and lubrication, were introduced, culminating in the introduction of the ultra-high-speed air rotor handpiece in the late 1950s.[5,6]

The result of these developments was that cavity preparation time was greatly reduced and patient comfort increased. However, as the restorative materials remained relatively unchanged, cavity designs did not change.[7] By the late 1960s the problems inherent in overextension of cavities were beginning to be recognized, and some of the leading educators were suggesting limitations. Unfortunately these recommendations coincided with the introduction of the ultra-high-speed cutting instruments, which so facilitated removal of tooth structure that it was very easy to overextend a cavity. Obviously the larger the cavity, the weaker the remaining tooth structure, and further problems began to be recognized in the form of split cusps and undue modification to occlusal anatomy[8,9] (Figs 4-1a and 4-1b). Overextension led to loss of esthetics as well as significant alterations to the occlusion.

During this period there were improvements in amalgam alloys and the methods of clinical handling.[10] The original alloy particles were cut by lathe, were relatively rough, and varied greatly in size. Improved manufacturing systems led to controlled grain size and eventually to the development of spherical particles that were easier to condense into the cavity. Capsulation of alloys was introduced, leading to superior control of the mixed material and the potential for higher-quality restorations.

In the absence of adhesion, the problems of retention remained contentious. Black maintained that additional retentive design elements were not required beyond straight flat parallel walls and sharp internal line angles. In the 1960s and 1970s Markley[11] and Outhwaite et al[12] introduced the use of threaded pins to enhance retention in larger cavities. Subsequently it was suggested that pins would reinforce the crown of the tooth and bind the cusps together.[13] Their use was then recommended even in relatively small cavities. The rather limited benefits of these systems soon became apparent, and they are now out of favor.

The benefits of retentive grooves and ditches have been debated since the early 1900s and are still discussed in the literature.[14–16] Certainly, unlike pins, they do not add any stress to the remaining crown of the tooth, and it is possible, with care, to embrace the central core of a badly broken-down crown and form a sound basis for a full-coverage restoration.[17,18]

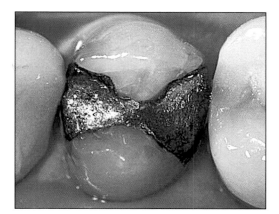

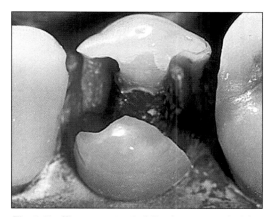

Fig 4-1a The maxillary first premolar was restored with amalgam using a G. V. Black cavity design. The buccal cusp remains exposed to heavy occlusal load, particularly if there is no canine rise in lateral excursion. It is therefore subject to splitting stresses and is now sensitive to pressure.

Fig 4-1b The same tooth following removal of the amalgam and modification of the cavity to provide a protective type of restoration. Note the split at the base of the buccal cusp that had led to pain on pressure during mastication.

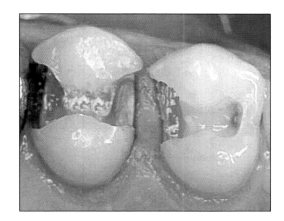

Fig 4-2 In spite of the fact that the carious lesions on the proximal surfaces of these teeth were relatively minor and had only just penetrated through the enamel, the standard G. V. Black–style cavities had to be prepared to enable placement of amalgam as the restorative material. The cavity margins were extended beyond the lesion as indicated by Black's theory that this would control the disease.

The most recent attempt to overcome the lack of adhesion with amalgam is to line the cavity with a bonding medium, such as resin or glass ionomer, and expect that to bind the cusps together.[13] Because these materials are used in a very thin section and the resins hydrolyze over time, they will not be strong in tension and the results should not be expected to be effective for the long term.[19]

The most significant aspect of all these changes is that they have been predicated on the continuing use of amalgam in the original G. V. Black cavity designs, possibly with minor modifications. When dealing with an initial lesion, regardless of the extent of the caries involvement, it was necessary to prepare a standard cavity design (Fig 4-2). It had to be deep enough to provide resistance form in the amalgam, wide enough to properly condense it, and extended far enough proximally to be in self-cleansing areas.[20] It was also necessary to remove all of the occlusal fissures because it is not possible to finish an amalgam margin in the middle of a fissure. At the time the classification was formulated, all these points were valid, but with the advent of adhesive restorative materials, this no longer holds true.

Adhesive Dentistry

In the late 1940s polymer chemistry became available to dentistry. Kramer and McLean[21] were among the first to try to show adhesion between resins and tooth structure, but the early attempts were not clinically successful. By the mid-1950s Buonocore[22] had shown that etching enamel would lead to a micromechanical attachment between enamel and a resin restoration, and this has proven to be effective and long lasting.[23] The strength of the union is limited only by the strength of the enamel. As with any change, it took some years for this concept to be adopted by the profession, in part because the earliest resin restorative materials were unfilled and therefore showed high shrinkage on curing, as well as a high wear factor.[24] The technology to incorporate sufficient filler particles[25] into a resin to make a satisfactory restorative material took another 10 years, so it was not until the mid-1960s that composites were available for clinical use. Their continuous development led to the so-called hybrid resin composites, which became available in the mid-1980s.[26] Since that time, the only change to this group of

materials has been to vary the type and size of the filler particles as well as the size distribution.

The understanding of the micromechanical adhesion of resin to enamel has now been thoroughly investigated and the technique standardized. The cavity margins need to be in fully mineralized enamel, well supported by healthy dentin, and slightly beveled to provide adhesion to the ends of the enamel rods rather than the long axis (Figs 4-3a and 4-3b). However, in spite of extensive research into adhesion, either chemical or micromechanical, between dentin and resin composite the ultimate goal remains elusive.[27] There is still no consensus on the technology, and it remains a difficult and complex clinical challenge with little sign of success. Currently it is postulated that it is possible to develop a combined chemical and micromechanical union. However, resin is anhydrous and tends to break down over time as a result of hydrolysis. This poses problems because of the presence of water both from dentin tubules and the oral environment, so it seems longevity of the bond cannot be assured. Great care in clinical placement is required, and it is recommended that placement always be carried out under rubber dam to ensure freedom from unwanted contamination.

In the mid-1970s true chemical ion-exchange adhesion to both enamel and dentin became available through the glass-ionomer materials.[28,29] These water-based materials survive well in the presence of water. Although the tooth structure is partially demineralized through caries, it is still possible to develop a union that will prevent microleakage and appears to be long lasting.[30] At the same

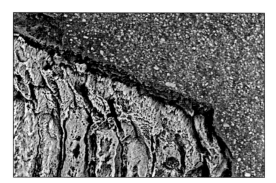

Fig 4-3a The occlusal margin of a resin composite restoration that has been lightly beveled so that adhesion can be gained through the ends of the enamel rods.

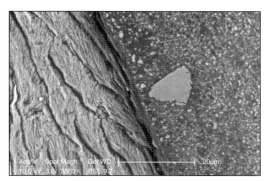

Fig 4-3b The same restoration showing the adaptation of the resin composite further down the vertical wall of the cavity. Note that the potential for micromechanical adhesion around the enamel rods is notably less because only the long axis of the rods is available.

time, this material is capable of taking part in an ion exchange with remaining tooth structure that will assist, to a degree, in remineralization and healing of a carious lesion even when the lesion is advanced.[31] Black maintained that it was necessary to remove all softened, demineralized dentin on the floor of the cavity, but it is now possible to remineralize and heal partly demineralized dentin in these areas.

With these two forms of adhesion, it should be possible to revise cavity designs and retain some of the natural tooth structure that had to be removed according to Black's standards. Now that the caries process is better understood, it is possible to control the disease to a considerable degree so that extension for prevention is no longer justified.[32] Neither is it necessary to provide for mechanical interlocking between tooth structure and restoration. Therefore, it is

suggested that, in dealing with new lesions, cavity design should be limited largely to the extent of the carious lesion.

Since both of the adhesive materials are tooth colored, there is an added incentive for the preservation of natural tooth structure. If all new lesions were restored with adhesive materials using minimal cavity designs,[18] then, over time, it is likely that the need for replacement dentistry would be reduced and the natural strength and esthetics of the tooth crown could be preserved substantially longer.

Caries Control

Because dental caries is a bacterial disease, the profession should not continue to attempt to control it through surgical removal of natural tooth structure. The involvement of bacteria has been acknowledged since the late 1880s,[1] but methods for control of caries have evolved slowly. The action of the fluoride ion within the oral environment has been better understood since the 1950s, so it has been possible to limit caries at a community level as well as for individuals.[33] The use of systemic fluoride through community water supplies, as well as the incorporation of fluoride in dentifrices, has reduced the intensity of caries in many populations, but at the individual level it is still a multifactorial disease. Specific infection control became possible following the advent of chlorhexidine in the 1970s.[34,35] Reduction in the frequency of intake of refined carbohydrates combined with regular oral hygiene routines are necessary corollaries for successful caries control, and it is up to the patient, to a large degree, to understand and control their own caries problem.

Placement of a restoration will only repair the damage caused by the disease, so it is necessary to control it before any surgical intervention is undertaken. There is no long-term gain from placing restorations without first controlling the caries because the disease will either continue or recur. Many surveys of restorative dentistry have cited recurrent caries as a cause of replacement dentistry and suggested that either the operator or the restorative material is at fault.[36] The real problem is the continuing presence of the original infection—or possibly reinfection at a later date. It must be accepted that no restorative material will prevent caries. However, poorly handled restorative materials will allow for a continuation of the problem. As long as the smooth surface of the crown or the integrity of the interface between a restoration and the cavity surface is

compromised, it will not be possible to completely control the bacterial flora, and the disease may continue. The most effective method of control is the maintenance of the smooth contours of the tooth crown combined with limitation of the bacterial flora.

Modifications to Cavity Designs

Once the disease is controlled, it is then possible to consider the problems posed by the damage to both the enamel and dentin resulting from caries. It is essential to restore the smooth form of the natural crown so that there will no longer be surface irregularities in which bacterial plaque can accumulate. All other natural surface defects, such as pits and fissures, can be sealed at the same time without necessarily involving them in surgical exploration.[37,38]

This discussion is related primarily to restoration of new lesions, because the operator is still free to choose the appropriate material to be placed and therefore the cavity outline form. Little can be done to improve the cavity form in replacement dentistry because the cavity was probably prepared according to the G. V. Black classification and was therefore designed initially for restoration with amalgam. This infers that, at this point, amalgam should not be abandoned as a restorative material because there will be pre-existing cavities that are too extensive to be restored, long term, with one of the adhesive materials.[39]

The basic rules laid down by Black for the preparation of a cavity included the need for access to the lesion.[40] This was

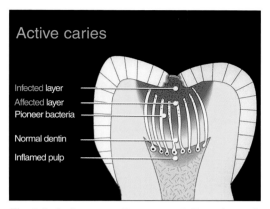

Fig 4-4 A diagrammatic representation of a carious lesion (after Massler[41]) showing the difference between the infected and the affected layers of carious dentin. The affected layer is demineralized but still retains the original form of the dentin tubules and is capable of being remineralized and healed. Therefore, there is no need to remove it, particularly if glass ionomer is to be used as the restorative material.

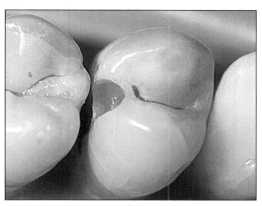

Fig 4-5 A "slot"-type minimal cavity design that is quite satisfactory when an adhesive restorative material is used. The design is limited to the removal of only the tooth structure that is beyond remineralization, thus retaining as much as possible the structural integrity of the crown of the tooth.

termed *convenience form*, and it is, of course, still necessary to open the lesion sufficiently to identify the extent of the problem. Black then defined the outline form of the cavity, which meant extending the cavity to a theoretically caries-free area—"extension for prevention." By modern standards it is only necessary to ensure removal of all infected tooth structure, and extension beyond that cannot be justified. That is to say, remove only enamel and dentin that are so broken down they are beyond remineralization and healing (Figs 4-4 and 4-5). Remaining tooth structure, even though it may be partially demineralized, can be retained and remineralized.

In the absence of adhesive materials, the next important factor is to provide mechanical interlocks between the restoration and the tooth—that is, to provide *retention form*. Now it is only necessary to develop a surface that is amenable to adhesion—chemical or micromechanical. Finally there is the need for resistance form in the restoration itself. In other words, the cavity has to be sufficiently deep for the restorative material to withstand occlusal loads. This is still essential because the presently used adhesive materials have lower physical properties than does amalgam.

Cavity Design for Resin Composite

At this time adhesion between tooth structure and resin composite is limited to micromechanical union with enamel only. It was shown by Buonocore[22] in the

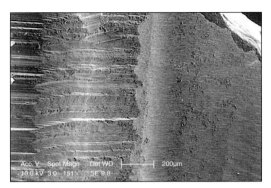

Fig 4-6 The vertical walls of this cavity were initially prepared with an 80-µm diamond bur, and the relatively rough surface is shown on the left. Subsequently the wall was polished with a 25-µm diamond bur, and the result, shown on the right, will allow far more efficient adaptation of an adhesive restorative material.

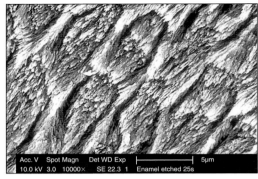

Fig 4-7 A scanning electron microscopic view of the ends of enamel rods showing the effect of etching. The enamel crystals have been removed to some extent from the enamel rods, allowing a degree of porosity and the ingress of an unfilled resin bond. (Courtesy of Dr Hien Ngo.)

1950s that etching enamel for a limited period with 37% orthophosphoric acid would dissolve the outer layers of the enamel rods and lead to a degree of porosity on the surface. This would allow the penetration of an unfilled resin up to 50 µm into the enamel, leading to a strong union between the two.[23]

The concept works best at the ends of the enamel rods rather than along the long axis, so it is desirable to slightly bevel the margins of the cavity. It is also important to rely on fully mineralized enamel that is supported with sound dentin and is free of microcracks. This may mean that, on occasion, the cavity should be extended in limited directions to reach enamel that is acceptable.

One of the basic requirements for good adhesion is that the adherend be applied to a smooth surface.[42] For a small new lesion, basic cavity preparation is best carried out with a tapered-cylinder diamond bur at intermediate high speed (60,000 to 80,000 rpm) under air-water spray. A diamond bur with an 80-µm grit will cut quickly and efficiently for the development of the initial access form, but the resultant surface will be relatively rough. This surface should then be lightly polished, at a slightly reduced speed, with a 25-µm grit diamond; the surface will then be smooth enough to accept adhesion[43] (Fig 4-6). With care the enamel will also be free of microcracks. A small round bur can then be used to remove remaining demineralized dentin, particularly around the walls. An appropriate lining should then be placed before the cavity is prepared for the resin composite. The enamel margins should then be etched. This will modify the surface tension to the extent that an unfilled, low-viscosity resin bonding agent will penetrate the enamel rods to a satisfactory level (Fig 4-7).

On the assumption that the disease is controlled, there will be no need for extension for prevention. However, as there is no water in resin composite, there can be no ion migration, either into or out of

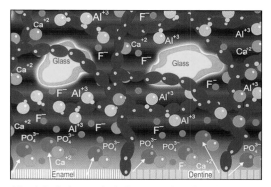

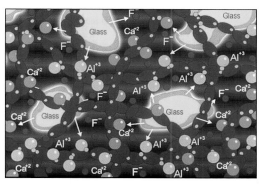

Fig 4-8 A theoretical diagram showing the development of the ion exchange between glass ionomer and the tooth surface. Note that the polyalkenoic acid chains actually penetrate the surface of both enamel and dentin and displace phosphate ions, releasing them into the cement. Each phosphate ion takes with it a calcium ion to maintain electrolytic balance, thus leading to an ion-enriched layer at the interface. As the acid is buffered by the release of the ions, the pH will rise and the interface will set as a new ion-enriched material between the tooth and the restoration.

Fig 4-9 A theoretical diagram of the acid-base setting reaction between the glass powder and the polyalkenoic acid. Note that only the surface of each particle is attacked by the acid, releasing calcium and aluminum ions as well as fluoride ions, which remain free and are not part of the matrix. The calcium polyacrylate chains form first, and then the aluminum polyacrylate chains follow immediately. There is also a halo of a siliceous hydrogel surrounding each of the glass particles, and it is thought that this will increase resistance to acid attack.

this material, and therefore bioactivity is not possible. This means that the cavity margins need to be extended to incorporate any area of enamel that is partly demineralized. Adjacent surface defects such as pits and fissures can be etched and sealed with an unfilled resin as part of the restorative procedures.

Cavity Design for Glass-Ionomer Cement

Adhesion between a glass ionomer and tooth structure is the result of an ion-exchange mechanism initiated by the dissolution of the tooth surface by the polyalkenoic acid contained in the cement[44] (Fig 4-8). The same chemical exchange will occur with both enamel and dentin and, even in the presence of par-

tially demineralized tooth structure, the action will still take place. The acid/base setting reaction of the glass ionomer will release calcium and aluminum ions from the glass particles (Fig 4-9). When the freshly mixed cement is applied to the tooth surface, the polyalkenoic acid will release phosphate ions, and each of these will take a calcium ion with it to maintain electrolytic balance. As more ions are released, the acid will be buffered, and a new ion-enriched material will develop at the interface between the restoration and the tooth. This appears to be strongly attached to both, and any future failure will be cohesive in the glass ionomer rather than adhesive at the interface. There is also evidence of a degree of chemical union between collagen and the glass ionomer.[45]

An additional advantage of glass ionomers is that, because they are water based, there is a potential for a continuing ion-exchange mechanism between the restoration and the tooth structure that appears to continue throughout the life of the restoration.[46] An ongoing fluoride release was identified when they were first introduced,[47] and a degree of resistance to further demineralization in the vicinity of a restoration has been attributed to this. It has been shown recently that both calcium and phosphate ions can also be released, and these can be of value in remineralization of partially demineralized enamel and dentin.[31]

Two surfaces of a restoration are significant to this ion exchange. There will be a continuing release of fluoride from the outer surface of a restoration, and this will be compensated by an uptake of calcium and hydroxyl ions from the saliva back into the cement. The fluoride will be taken up to some extent by the surrounding enamel, and the other ions will help to reinforce and mature the outer surface of the restoration. The inner surface of a glass-ionomer restoration, directly in contact with the dentin, will also release calcium, aluminum, and fluoride ions as long as the pH of the surrounding interface is low. The pH of the polyalkenoic acid is in the vicinity of 1.9, which will account for the release of ions from the dentin as well. As the pH is buffered by the release of ions, the material will set, but in the meantime there will have been a considerable ion release and they will penetrate deeply from the glass ionomer into the demineralized dentin. This potential for remineralization suggests that it is not necessary to remove all softened dentin from the floor of a cavity.

This ability to facilitate healing and remineralization within the dentin is valuable and suggests that glass ionomer is probably the ideal base for any restoration. The only limitation at this time is its relatively low resistance to fracture, which means that, in a larger restoration, it may need to be overlaid or protected by another restorative material.

Resulting from the above, it is suggested that only limited-access form is required for a glass-ionomer restoration. There is no need to extend to the outer margin of demineralized enamel because, provided that the tooth surface is smooth and capable of remineralization, it is likely that the uptake of ions will be sufficient to repair the surface and heal it. For the same reason, there would appear to be no need to remove all demineralized dentin from the floor of a cavity. As long as there is clean enamel and dentin around the periphery, the underlying areas will be fully sealed through the ion-exchange adhesion. Remaining bacteria will then become dormant.[31]

The small tapered-cylinder diamond, with 80-μm grit, recommended for preparing a resin composite cavity is also suitable under these circumstances and, when used at intermediate high speed under air-water spray, it is unlikely to cause microcracks in surrounding enamel. The walls should be polished with a 25-μm diamond bur to enhance adaptation of the cement. Because it is necessary only to remove the enamel and dentin that is incapable of remineralization, the extent of the cavity can be limited. The walls should be cleaned back to sound dentin with a small round bur, and the cavity is ready to be conditioned. Pits and fissures and other defects in adjacent tooth structure can be sealed against future caries without any surgical intervention.[48]

Conditioning with 10% polyacrylic acid for 10 seconds will remove the smear layer and modify the surface tension to the extent that the cement will adapt readily and the ion-exchange adhesion will be enhanced. The only limitation to the use of glass ionomer at this time seems to be the inherent brittleness of the material, although this can be overcome by laminating over it with another stronger material, such as amalgam or resin composite.

Changes in Operative Dentistry

The changes that have occurred over the last 100 years have been outlined above and attention is drawn to the fact that the only area that has not changed is basic cavity design. Improved methods for control of the disease mean that the concept of trying to eliminate a bacterial disease through surgery is no longer tenable. Methods of cavity preparation have changed considerably, to the extent that a carious lesion is relatively simple to access. Reliable adhesion between the tooth structure and the restoration eliminates the need to remove more tooth structure for the development of retentive elements. The advent of a bioactive material that will assist in the remineralization of that part of the tooth that is not completely demineralized means that even more tooth structure can be safely conserved.

A number of published papers have recommended modifications to cavity design that take into account the benefits of adhesion as well as ion exchange.

The concepts offered encourage preservation of tooth structure with maintenance of esthetics and strength in the remaining tooth crown.[49–52]

In light of this, it is suggested that the next change in operative dentistry should be recognition that the extent of the cavities that have to be prepared for restoration of a tooth crown damaged by a prolonged attack of caries can be limited. By limiting the amount of tooth structure removed, it will be possible to retain much of the natural strength of the crown as well as of the original occlusal anatomy. This in turn will increase the potential life span of restorations and reduce the need for replacements. It may also minimize the problems of split cusps. At the same time, natural esthetics will be retained and the problems posed by the need to maintain or restore the original appearance will be limited.

However, one of the barriers to change is the continuing use of the G. V. Black system of cavity classification. It is based on the preparation of a standard cavity design, developed for restoration with amalgam, and does not take into account the elimination of caries through control of the bacterial flora.

A modified classification has been proposed that recognizes the presence of carious lesions instead of defining specific cavities. It identifies the lesion from the very earliest stage in which it should be able to be controlled and healed with no surgical procedures. It follows the development of a lesion in stages up to the point where the tooth is extensively damaged, and each stage can be identified and recorded in detail. Further information can be found in the literature, but the framework is explained here for emphasis.[42,53,54]

Table 4-1 Modified classification of cavity design*

Site	No Cavity 0	Minimal 1	Moderate 2	Enlarged 3	Extensive 4
Pit/fissure 1	1.0	1.1	1.2	1.3	1.4
Contact area 2	2.0	2.1	2.2	2.3	2.4
Cervical area 3	3.0	3.1	3.2	3.3	3.4

*Reprinted from Mount and Hume[52] with permission.

Classification for Minimal Intervention Dentistry

This classification has been developed to recognize carious lesions at different stages. The system has been designed so that it can be used successfully for replacement dentistry as well as minimal intervention.

It is suggested that only three sites on the crown of a tooth are likely to become carious as a result of plaque accumulation (Table 4-1). It is also recognized that a cavity, if untreated, is likely to progress from the earliest stage at which, with care, it can be remineralized, to the point at which the tooth crown is badly broken down. These stages should be able to be identified and recorded because methods of treatment and selection of materials are likely to vary as the lesion enlarges.

Lesion Site

Carious lesions occur in only three different sites on the surface of a tooth crown.

Site 1—The pits and fissures on the occlusal surface of posterior teeth and other defects on otherwise smooth enamel surfaces

Site 2—The contact areas between any two teeth, anterior or posterior

Site 3—The cervical areas related to the gingival tissues, including exposed root surfaces

Lesion Size

A neglected lesion will continue to extend as an area of demineralization in relation to one of the sites noted above. As it extends, the complexities of restoration will increase. The sizes that can be readily identified are as follows:

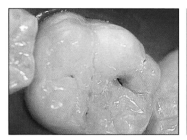
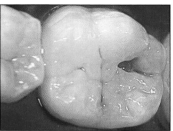
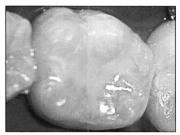

Fig 4-10a A site 1, size 1 lesion on the occlusal surface of a mandibular molar. There is a carious lesion in the distal fissure and some apparent demineralization in parts of the other fissures. Some level of surgical intervention is required before restoration.

Fig 4-10b The surgical intervention has been limited to the frank caries only. The cavity, along with the rest of the occlusal fissure system, will be restored with a glass-ionomer cement.

Fig 4-10c The glass ionomer has been placed and will act as both a restoration and a fissure sealant. The intrinsic strength of the crown of the tooth has been maintained. Only a minimal amount of restorative material is exposed to occlusal load and can therefore be expected to last a long time.

Size 0—The initial lesion at any site that can be identified but has not yet resulted in surface cavitation; healing may be possible.

Size 1—The smallest minimal lesion requiring operative intervention. The cavity is just beyond healing through remineralization.

Size 2—A moderate-sized cavity. There is still sufficient sound tooth structure to maintain the integrity of the remaining crown and accept the occlusal load.

Size 3—The cavity needs to be modified and enlarged to provide some protection for the remaining crown against the occlusal load. A split already exists at the base of a cusp, or, if the cusp is not protected, a split is likely to develop.

Size 4—The cavity is extensive, following loss of a cusp from a posterior tooth or an incisal edge from an anterior tooth.

As an illustration of minimal intervention operative dentistry, Figs 4-10a to 4-10c show the treatment of a small lesion in the distal fissure of a mandibular first molar. Clinical examination suggests that there is some dentin involvement below the fissure in the enamel. However, it is limited in extent, and there appears to be no indication for the full removal of the rest of the fissure system as suggested by Black. Minimal surgical intervention is recommended to determine the extent of the problem. Having defined the size of the lesion it is sufficient to restore it with a high-strength glass ionomer while at the same time sealing the remainder of the system with the same adhesive cement. Such restorations show a very acceptable longevity.

Conservative treatment of a minimal proximal lesion is also highly desirable. Maintenance of the integrity of the marginal ridge will sustain the overall

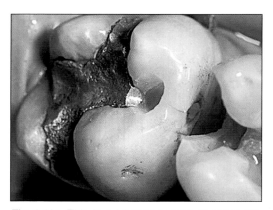

Fig 4-11a This is a laboratory case showing the essential elements of a "tunnel" cavity. The original lesion can be seen on the proximal surface of the tooth, and entry through the enamel is limited. The occlusal approach through a limited tunnel can be seen, and the marginal ridge remains intact, thus maintaining the strength of the crown as much as possible.

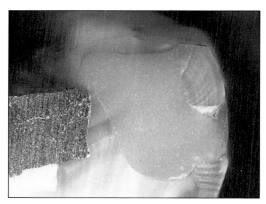

Fig 4-11b The restored tooth has been sectioned mesiodistally through the restoration. The extent of the carious penetration can be seen. Note that not all demineralized enamel was removed from the proximal surface because what remains is expected to remineralize and heal in the presence of the glass ionomer.

strength of the crown of the tooth and limit the potential for development of splits at the base of a cusp. Figures 4-11a and 4-11b suggest the value of this approach. The amount of occlusal surface involved is limited, and the proximal lesion need not be extended further than the area of actual cavitation. Figure 4-11b shows a cross-section of the restored tooth following restoration with glass ionomer. Note that there are still limited areas of demineralized enamel surrounding the restoration on the proximal enamel, but, as the surface is smooth, the enamel is expected to remineralize and heal in the presence of the ion release from the glass ionomer.

There are many variations in cavity design available when using the adhesive restorative materials, and the concept of "extension for prevention" no longer needs to be applied. It is only necessary to eliminate surface cavitation to prevent further plaque accumulation and then to ensure that the cavity margins are sealed against further bacterial invasion.

Conclusions

The only real constant in life is change, and dentistry is no exception. In the past 100 years there has been considerable change in methods for caries control, equipment, techniques, and materials, but in spite of this, there has been one constant in this profession—the G. V. Black system of cavity classification. While there was no valid reason or justification for change for the first 75 years, the advent of long-term adhesion, and now a bioactive restorative material, offers a serious challenge to the profession and opens the way for change.

If modern restorative materials are to be used properly to achieve optimum results, then it is essential that the approach to treatment become disease oriented rather than remain focused on cavity design. Caries cannot be cured by surgery, but surgery is required once the tooth is irrevocably damaged by the disease. Now, with adhesion and bioactive materials, surgery can be limited because minimal intervention will help to retain both the strength and esthetics of each tooth. The adoption of a new classification for carious lesions will help to overcome the psychologic barrier to change.

References

1. Miller WD. The etiology of dental caries. Independent Pract (Dent) 1883:4.

2. Black GV. A Work on Operative Dentistry. Vol 2: The Technical Procedures in Filling Teeth. Chicago: Medico-Dental, 1917:137.

3. Walsh JP. Critical view of cutting instruments in cavity preparation 1: Diamond stones. Int Dent J 1953;4:36–41.

4. Lammie GA. A study of some different tungsten carbide burs. Dent Rec 1952;72:285–300.

5. Hartley JL, Amsterdam M, Ingraham R. Ultraspeed instrumentation for atraumatic removal of tooth structure. J Am Acad Gold Foil Oper 1971;14:16–18.

6. Peyton FA. Status report on dental operating handpieces. J Am Dent Assoc 1974;89:1162.

7. Ingraham R. Application of sound biomechanical principles in the design of inlay, amalgam and gold foil restorations. J Am Dent Assoc 1950;40:402–413.

8. Cavel WT, Kelsey WP, Blankenau RJ. An in vivo study of cuspal fracture. J Prosthet Dent 1985; 53:38–42.

9. Ferguson NC. Fractured cusps. J Am Acad Gold Foil Oper 1972;15:19–24.

10. Greener EH. Amalgam—yesterday, today and tomorrow. Oper Dent 1979;4:24–35.

11. Markley MR. Pin-retained and pin-reinforced amalgam. J Am Dent Assoc 1966;73:1295–1300.

12. Outhwaite WC, Garman TA, Pashley DH. Pin vs. slot retention in extensive amalgam restorations. J Prosthet Dent 1979;41:369–400.

13. Summitt JB, Osborne JW. Amalgam restorations. In: Summitt JB, Robbins JW, Schwartz RS (eds). Fundamentals of Operative Dentistry: A Contemporary Approach. Chicago: Quintessence, 2001:306–364.

14. Rodda JC. Modern Class II amalgam cavity preparations. New Zealand Dent J 1972;68: 132–138.

15. Wilson RA, Fiocca VL. Current concepts in cavity design for amalgam restorations. Ill Dent J 1975;44:275–278.

16. Birtcil RF, Venton EA. Extra-coronal amalgam restorations utilizing available tooth structure for retention. J Prosthet Dent 1976;35:171–178.

17. Mount GJ. The use of amalgam to protect remaining tooth structure. New Zealand Dent J 1977;73:15–20.

18. Mount GJ, Hume WR. Preservation and Restoration of Tooth Structure. London: Mosby, 1998:59–61.

19. Hawthorne W, Smales R, Webster D. Long-term survival of restorative materials in private practice [abstract 85]. J Dent Res 1994;73:747.

20. Markley MR. Silver amalgam. Oper Dent 1984; 9:10–25.

21. Kramer IRH, McLean JW. Alterations in the staining reaction of dentine resulting from a constituent of a self-polymerising resin. Br Dent J 1952;93:150–153.

22. Buonocore M. A simple method of increasing the adhesion of acrylic filling materials to enamel surfaces. J Dent Res 1955;34:849–853.

23. Jorgensen KD, Shimokobe H. Adaptation of resinous restorative materials to acid-etched enamel surfaces. Scand J Dent Res 1975;83:31–36.

24. Nealon FG. Acrylic restorations: Operative nonpressure procedure. J Prosthet Dent 1952;2: 513–518.

25. Bowen RL. Properties of a silica-reinforced polymer for dental restorations. J Am Dent Assoc 1963;66:57–60.

26. Phillips RW (ed). Science of Dental Materials, ed 9. Philadelphia: Saunders, 1991:229–233.

27. Phillips RW (ed). Science of Dental Materials, ed 9. Philadelphia: Saunders, 1991:238–241.

28. Kent BE, Wilson AD. The properties of a glass-ionomer cement. Br Dent J 1973;135:322–326.

29. Wilson AD, McLean JW. Glass-Ionomer Cement. London: Quintessence, 1989.

30. Mount GJ. Adhesion of glass-ionomer cement in the clinical environment. Oper Dent 1991;16:141–148.

31. Ngo H, Marino V, Mount GJ. Calcium, strontium, aluminum, sodium and fluoride release from four glass-ionomers [abstract 75]. J Dent Res 1998;77:641.

32. Walsh LJ. Preventive dentistry for the general practitioner. Aust Dent J 2000;45:76–82.

33. Silverstone LM. The effect of fluoride in the remineralisation of enamel caries and caries-like lesions in vitro. J Public Health Dent 1982;24:42–53.

34. Bowden G. Mutans streptococci, caries and chlorhexidene. J Can Dent Assoc 1996;62:700–707.

35. Loesche WJ. Clinical and microbiological aspects of chemotherapeutic agents used according to the specific plaque hypothesis. J Dent Res 1979;58:2404–2412.

36. Mjör IA. Glass-ionomer restorations and secondary caries: A preliminary report. Quintessence Int 1996;27:171–174.

37. Simonsen RJ. Retention and effectiveness of dental sealant after 15 years. J Am Dent Assoc 1991;122:34–42.

38. Going RE, Loesche WJ, Grainger DA, Syed SA. The viability of microorganisms in carious lesions 5 years after covering with a fissure sealant. J Am Dent Assoc 1978;97:455–462.

39. Shillingburg HT, Jacobi R, Brackett SE. Preparation modifications for damaged vital posterior teeth. Dent Clin North Am 1985;29:305–326.

40. Black GV. Operative Dentistry, vol 3. Treatment of Caries. Chicago: Medico-Dental, 1948:145–158.

41. Massler M. Preventive endodontics: Vital pulp therapy. Dent Clin North Am 1967 Nov:663–673.

42. Glanz PO. Adhesion to teeth. Int Dent J 1977;27:324–332.

43. Mount GJ. An Atlas of Glass-Ionomer Cements: A Clinician's Guide, ed 3. London: Martin Dunitz, 2001.

44. Akinmade AO, Nicholson JW. Review—Glass-ionomer cements as adhesives. Part 1. Fundamental aspects and their clinical relevance. J Mater Sci Mater Med 1993;4:95–101.

45. Akinmade A. Adhesion of glass-polyalkenoate cement to collagen [abstract 633]. J Dent Res 1994;73(special issue):181.

46. Ngo H, Biological potential of glass-ionomers. In: Mount GJ. An Atlas of Glass-Ionomer Cements. London: Martin Dunitz, 2002:43–55.

47. Forsten L. Fluoride release and uptake by glass-ionomers and related materials and its clinical effect. Biomaterials 1998;19:503–508.

48. McLean JW, Wilson AD. Fissure sealing and filling with an adhesive glass-ionomer cement. Br Dent J 1974;136:269–276.

49. Jinks GM. Fluoride impregnated cements and their effect on the activity of interproximal caries. J Dent Child 1963;30:87–92.

50. Knight GM. The use of adhesive materials in the conservative restoration of selected posterior teeth. Aust Dent J 1984;29:324–331.

51. Morand J-M, Jonas P. Resin-modified glass-ionomer cement restorations of posterior teeth with proximal carious lesions. Quintessence Int 1995;26:389–394.

52. Mount GJ. Minimal treatment of the carious lesion. Int Dent J 1991;16:141–148.

53. Mount GJ, Hume WR. A revised classification of carious lesions by site and size. Quintessence Int 1997;28:301–303.

54. Roulet J-F, Degrange M. Adhesion: The Silent Revolution in Dentistry. Chicago: Quintessence, 1999.

Chapter 5

Diagnosis and Restoration of Proximal Carious Lesions

Götz M. Lösche

Abstract

Caries detection and diagnosis, and subsequent restoration, in proximal areas are challenging for restorative dentists. For an accurate diagnosis, visual and tactile examination should be supplemented with evaluation of bitewing radiographs or the use of an orthodontic separating rubber band, an intraoral camera with or without an endoscope, and interdental impressions. All of these tools are effective for improving diagnosis at an early stage. Minimally invasive treatment should then follow. Various cavity preparations and treatment methods are discussed.

Dentistry has changed as we have learned that caries per se is not irreversible but can be stopped and reversed with adequate prophylactic therapy. Complete restoration, however, is only possible when the carious lesion is limited to the enamel surface. Therefore, the goal of dentistry should be the detection of caries at the earliest stage possible to allow remineralization of the lesion, to prevent progression of the lesion, or to intervene with minimally invasive therapy.

Occlusal Carious Lesions

For occlusal sites this goal has almost been achieved. In countries with relatively high caries prevalence, sealing of the occlusal fissure system has proved to be an adequate tool to minimize the caries risk in patients with high caries activity.[1] Regarding the retention rates of preventive fissure sealants, the efficacy of this therapy is obvious.[2-5] It is important to keep in mind, however, that many long-term results have been achieved with chemically curing sealants that showed deep penetration into the acid-etch pattern of the enamel. With light-curing sealants penetration depth is highly dependent on the time from application to curing.[6] As long as the adhesive bond is intact, underestimated, or deliberately sealed, carious lesions should not present a problem, since sealed restorations have proved to prevent the progression of caries in dentin over a long period of time.[7]

Fissure caries can be diagnosed by measuring the electric resistance (Electronic Caries Monitor, Lode Diagnostics, Groningen, The Netherlands) or by using a probe based on laser fluorescence (DIAGNOdent, KaVo, Biberach, Germany). The diagnostic value of these techniques is superior to that of visual inspection or radiographic analysis. However, due to the high sensitivity, combined with a specificity substantially less than 100%, false-positive outcomes will occur, which is rather problematic. (Sensitivity is defined as the ability of a procedure to find the diseased subjects among a population. Specificity is the ability of a procedure to find the healthy subjects among a population.) Therefore, these sophisticated tools should not be used without careful consideration. These instruments are valuable, but taking into account their low specificity (cfr supra), they should be used in conjunction with the clinical investigation to formulate the diagnosis.[8,9]

If a clinician decides to open a questionable fissure as a second step in the minimally invasive strategy, the use of small, flame-shaped diamond burs is highly recommended, because these are the least invasive. The resulting cavity preparations are so small that they can be easily filled using a total-etch technique and a flowable composite. If the lesions are larger, due to caries, then the use of a small-particle hybrid composite is advocated.

The most innovative, noninvasive procedure for caries treatment is ozone treatment, in which the carious fissure system or the softened lesion is selectively subjected to ozone (HealOzone, CurOzone, Aurora, Ontario, Canada) (see chapter 7), which kills the pathogenic bacteria. The demineralized areas are remineralized in a second step. If this approach, which has shown promising results in short-term scientific studies,[10] is to be successful in the long term, clinical use must be documented with carefully designed clinical studies.

Proximal Carious Lesions

Treatment of a carious lesion is much more difficult in the proximal areas of posterior teeth. Lesions in these areas in most cases are slightly below the contact point and thus very difficult to assess with tactile and visual inspection (Fig 5-1). Therefore, bitewing radiographs are necessary for the diagnosis of proximal caries in posterior teeth. These radiographs allow definite and clear recommendations for therapeutic procedures if the lesion is limited to enamel (D1—the lesion is in the outer half of the enamel layer, D2—the lesion is up to the dentino-enamel junction [DEJ]) and also if the lesion is deep into dentin, ie, between the middle of the dentin and the pulp (D4) (Fig 5-2).[11] For lesions located in the outer half of the dentin (D3), it is difficult to determine the best treatment because no macroscopic cavitation is present at the outer surface in about 50% of these lesions.[12–14] If the surface is intact (macroscopic), remineralization is possible in these cases.[15–16] If the decision to use invasive treatment is postponed for too long, whether due to underestimating the size of the lesion, misjudging the individual caries risk, or poor compliance of the patient, may lead to a situation in which a caries lesion that was originally small extends to the DEJ.[17] This situation is problematic for the reconstruction, even with the use of adhesive technology.[18–20]

Diagnostics and Therapy Decision

A study performed at the Department of Operative and Preventive Dentistry and Endodontics of the Charité (Berlin,

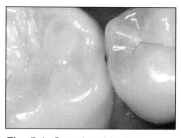

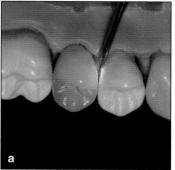

Fig 5-1 Questionable lesion on the proximal surface of a first molar.

| Caries monitoring | Yes | Yes | Yes/No | No |
| Invasive therapy | No | No | No/Yes | Yes |

Fig 5-2 Indications for caries monitoring and invasive therapy.

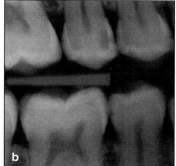
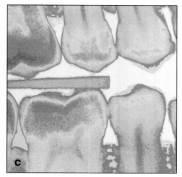

Fig 5-3 Procedures investigated for diagnosing the depth of proximal caries. *(a)* Fiber-optic transillumination (FOTI); *(b)* conventional radiograph; *(c)* digital radiograph.

Germany) may demonstrate how difficult it is to diagnose carious lesions that have barely reached the dentin (Rohwedder D, unpublished data, 1999). Twenty-four clinicians were asked to diagnose carious lesions with fiber-optic transillumination (FOTI) and conventional and digital radiographs (Digora, Soredex, Helsinki, Finland) (Fig 5-3). The teeth to be diagnosed were inserted into models with soft silicone gingiva to simulate the clinical situation and contained the following situations: small cavity (< 0.5 mm), large cavity (> 1 mm), white spot lesion (surface intact), brown spot lesion (surface intact), no lesion (control). The in vitro model was used so that the diagnosis could be validated with histologic sections.

In evaluating the sensitivity of the diagnostic procedures (Fig 5-4), it is obvious that both radiographic techniques were significantly superior to FOTI. For the diagnosis of dentin lesions, which were all in the outer half of the dentin (R3), the conventional radiographic technique was superior to FOTI and digital radiography. This may be explained by the lower resolution and sharpness of the digital radiographic image in comparison to the conventional one.[21] The results found in this study using the Digora system may be applied to other digital radiographic techniques.[22]

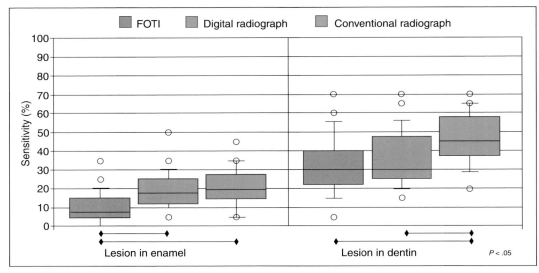

Fig 5-4 Sensitivity of tests shown in Fig 5-3.

It is notable that even with the most accurate technique, the conventional radiograph, only about 50% of the lesions were detected. This confirms the result of a meta-analysis of caries diagnosis with bitewing radiographs.[23] In this study, data of 1,700 proximal surfaces displayed with bitewing radiographs were analyzed. Only 50% of the caries surfaces were correctly diagnosed.[23] Knowing this diagnostic problem, one can easily understand and explain why there is a poor interexaminer agreement in diagnostic studies.[24-29] The use of software to reduce the variability of the diagnostic outcome has been successful.[30-32] Therefore, it seems reasonable to use computers for the therapy decision.[33]

The low specificity for the diagnosis of lesions limited to enamel (Fig 5-5) may be explained by frequent underestimation of the lesion. There was no single decision in which a lesion limited to enamel was falsely diagnosed as being in dentin. The diagnosis "dentinal caries" was correct in 96% of the cases. This high specificity, coupled with a high sensitivity, is proof of the fact that the size of the lesion is underestimated, rather than overestimated—an observation that was confirmed by other researchers.[16,34]

In the present study, the examiners were asked to make a treatment decision. None wanted to do this based on the FOTI or radiographic data alone. All clinicians wanted to correlate their findings with clinical inspection of the proximal surfaces. This procedure makes sense, since studies have shown that neither FOTI[35] nor radiographic findings alone[36,37] allow the conclusion that there is a lesion in the proximal surface.

The most effective procedure for an inspection of the proximal surface is the placement of an orthodontic separating rubber band (Fig 5-6) to open the interdental space.[14,38] After a few days, the rubber band can be removed and a wedge placed, allowing thorough inspection of the proximal surfaces. This separation of proximal surfaces not only allows a reliable

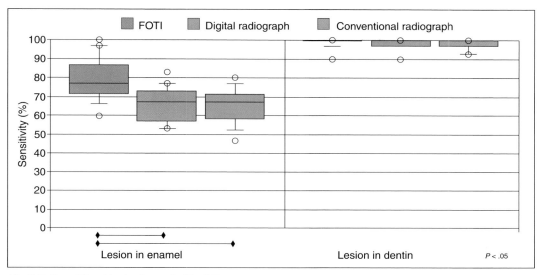

Fig 5-5 Specifity of tests shown in Fig 5-3.

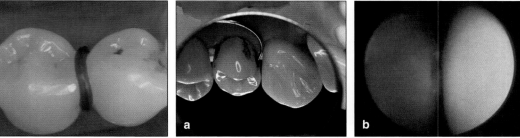

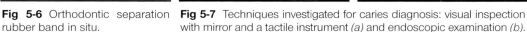

Fig 5-6 Orthodontic separation rubber band in situ.

Fig 5-7 Techniques investigated for caries diagnosis: visual inspection with mirror and a tactile instrument *(a)* and endoscopic examination *(b)*.

diagnosis, but it is advantageous in the event that an invasive procedure (restoration) is needed. With better accessibility, the cavity shape and the finishing and polishing process are optimized.[39] Therefore, the recall appointment should be set so that, if necessary, an adhesive restoration can be placed right away. However, this might be a burden for the office organization and the patient, which may explain why this excellent procedure is not widely used among practicing clinicians.

There is a definite need for a quick solution to diagnose small cavities in the interproximal area. A possible solution would be the use of an endoscope, an accessory tool available for many intraoral cameras. In order to determine if the endoscope would be a viable diagnostic tool, the 24 examiners of the previous study (Rohwedder D, unpublished data, 1999) were supplied with an endoscope to evaluate the same lesions (Fig 5-7). None of the examiners had experience using an endoscope

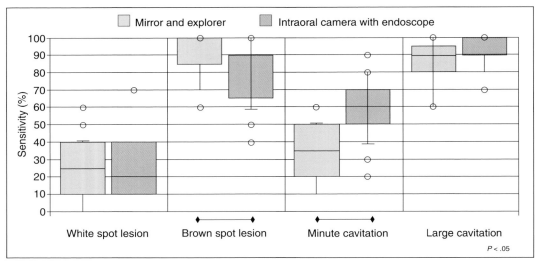

Fig 5-8 Sensitivity of the techniques shown in Fig 5-7.

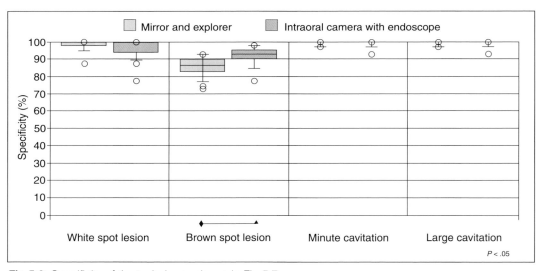

Fig 5-9 Specificity of the techniques shown in Fig 5-7.

for caries diagnosis; therefore, handling and interpretation problems could not be excluded. With the endoscope, the sensitivity of the diagnostic procedure, especially for small lesions, was found to be significantly improved. The improvement in the diagnosis of larger lesions, however, was seen only as a trend. Despite the higher sensitivity, there were no false-positive results (Figs 5-8 and 5-9). In a follow-up study in which the endoscope was compared with a common intraoral camera,

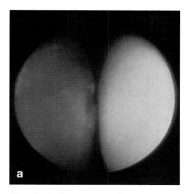
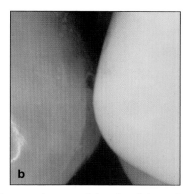

Fig 5-10 Small cavitation as seen with an endoscope *(a)* and an intraoral camera *(b)*.

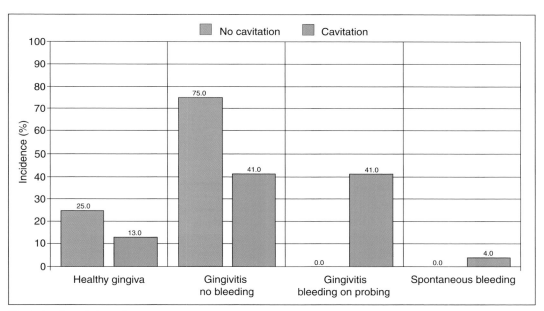

Fig 5-11 Correlation of bleeding on probing and the presence of proximal caries. Based on data from Ratledge et al.[40]

the results showed that the intraoral camera was not inferior to the endoscope, but was much easier to handle (Fig 5-10) (Lösche GM, unpublished data, 2002).

Since lesions on smooth surfaces are associated with higher plaque retention, it makes sense that in 41% of proximal surfaces with lesions, bleeding on probing was found. This fact can be used as an additional diagnostic hint (Fig 5-11).[40]

Another technique to evaluate the surface condition in especially narrow inter-

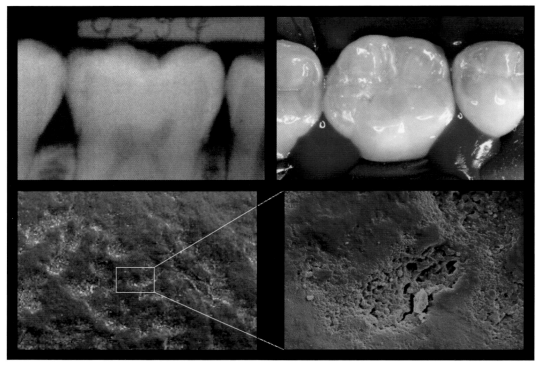

Fig 5-12 Use of impression material to evaluated questionable proximal surfaces.

dental spaces is to make an impression with a light-body silicone impression material injected into the interproximal area. With this technique it is possible to have a direct view of the surface, even under magnification (Fig 5-12).[41,42] The cleaning and removal of superficial organic deposits prior to impression making must be done with Superfloss (Oral-B, Boston, MA) and sodium hypochlorite. It is important to carefully dry the area before making the impression because silicones are hydrophobic materials.

Impedance spectroscopy compensating for the shortcomings of electric resistance measurement (polarization effects when d.c. or single-low-frequency a.c. currents are used) by measuring imped-

ance over a large range of frequencies was introduced in 1996 and showed 100% correlation[43] or almost perfect correspondence[44] between a.c. impedance measurements and the actual extent of the caries lesion on proximal surfaces in vitro.

Therapy of Proximal Carious Lesions

Looking at the clinically intact surface of an R3 carious lesion (caries has progressed histologically into the first half of the dentin) at high magnification (Fig 5-13), clinicians should realize that the therapy decision must not be made without careful consideration of the individual caries risk of the patient. It is known that microlesions

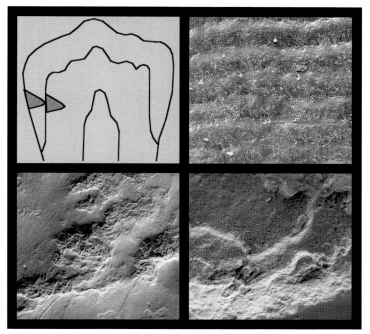

Fig 5-13 Surface morphology of D3 lesions, which are diagnosed by tactical and visual means as having an intact surface.

with active caries (Fig 5-13, bottom right) may be at least partially remineralized with intensive prevention and fluoridation and thus can be converted into inactive lesions (Fig 5-13, bottom left). If a white spot lesion is present in a patient with poor compliance and high caries risk, the clinician should implement invasive treatment even if the surface seems clinically intact.[11]

Restoration with internal access to a carious lesion

Removal of a macroscopically intact surface lesion to place a restoration is questionable for two reasons. First, it is contrary to the principles of minimally invasive dentistry, and, second, it is known that during the preparation of a proximal box the adjacent teeth are often (49% to 60%)[45] or almost always (90%[46]; 95% to 100%[47]) injured iatrogenically.

Therefore, different cavity preparation designs were proposed for teeth with intact or mostly intact proximal surface morphology (Fig 5-14). It was usually recommended to fill such "tunnel preparations" with silver-reinforced polyalkenoate cements (eg, Ketac Silver, 3M ESPE, Seefeld, Germany). Looking at the multitude of clinical studies dealing with this technique, one will note that the primary reason for failure is the fracture of the proximal ridge of the tooth or caries.[48] The reasons for failure are interconnected: the thickness of the marginal ridge is known to be critical for the sta-

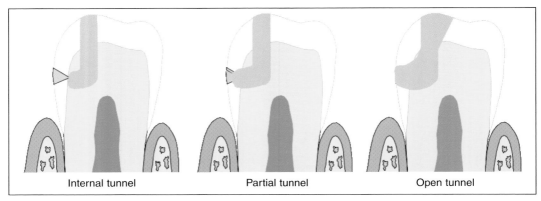

Fig 5-14 Three types of tunnel preparations.

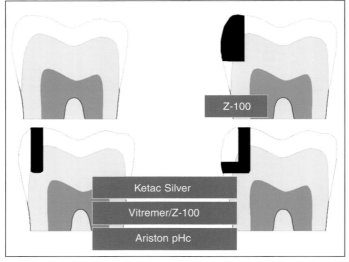

Fig 5-15 Experimental groups for the investigation on load bearing of tunnel cavity preparations restored with adhesive techniques.

bility if the preparation is filled with polyalkenoate cement (the thicker the ridge, the stronger the restoration).[49] However, the precision of caries removal is not so good if the remaining marginal ridge is thick[50,51] and the access to the lesion is small.[52] Because of this dilemma, it is recommended that tunnel preparations be limited to small lesions in pa-

tients with low or moderate caries activity.[53–55]

In another situation, considering that vertical access to the lesion is preferred over oblique access from the occlusal surface, leaving a very thick marginal ridge,[51] and considering that with sufficient caries excavation the dentin in the DEJ will be mostly removed,[56] a different

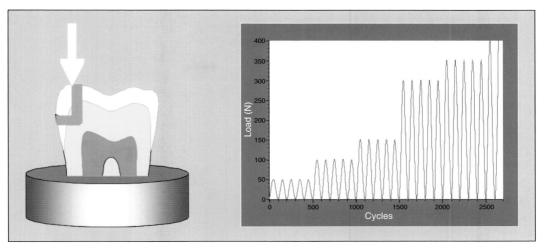

Fig 5-16 Principle of cyclic loading to failure.

treatment approach is needed. In this case, it is recommended to design a cavity with vertical access, through dentin, following the DEJ but to leave the proximal enamel as a cavity wall (Fig 5-15, bottom left). This enamel wall might then be stabilized "internally" with the adhesive technique.

To test this concept, the following experiment (Fig 5-15) was performed (Lösche GM, unpublished data, 2001). Thirty internal and open tunnel restorations each were used to form experimental groups (n = 10). The restorations were prepared with the following materials:

- Ketac Silver (3M ESPE)
- Vitremer/Z-100 + Scotchbond MP (3M ESPE)
- Ariston pHc + Ariston Liner (Ivoclar Vivadent, Schaan, Liechtenstein)

Ketac Silver was chosen because it is the material most often used for filling of tunnel restorations and can therefore be regarded as the gold standard. Vitremer was chosen for this indication because of its high fluoride-release potential,[57] its caries-protective effect[58] and its ability to remineralize initial carious lesions.[59] Ariston pHc was selected because of the manufacturer's claim of caries protection. It was applied according to the manufacturer's instructions in combination with the self-etching primer-adhesive.

There were two control groups. One included intact teeth and the other included teeth with proximal box preparations that were filled with the combination of Scotchbond MP and Z-100.

The samples were stored for 6 months in water and then submitted to cyclic stress (Fig 5-16). The marginal ridge was loaded intermittently with 2 Hz. The initial load was 1 to 50 N, and after every 500 cycles, the load was increased by 50 N for the next 500 cycles until the restora-

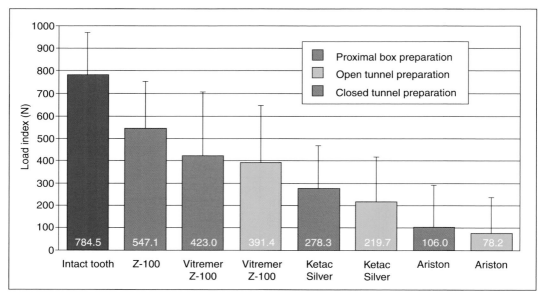

Fig 5-17 Load to fracture of tunnel restorations.

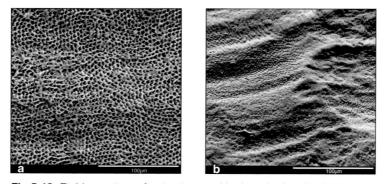

Fig 5-18 Etching pattern after treatment with phosphoric acid: *(a)* beveled enamel; *(b)* axial enamel from the inner side of an internal tunnel preparation.

tion or the tooth failed. A failure index was calculated from the raw data based on the following formula:

$$FI = L_1 \times n + L_2 \times n + L_3 \times n \dots + L_{max} \times n_{failure}$$

(FI = failure index; L = load; n = number of cycles; L_{max} = load when fail occurred; $n_{failure}$ = number of cycles with maximum load)

As seen in Fig 5-17 the intact teeth were able to withstand the highest load, which was significantly superior to all other groups. There was no significant difference between the proximal box preparation and the adhesive tunnel preparation. However, the tunnel preparations tended to show inferior results. The lack of stability may be explained

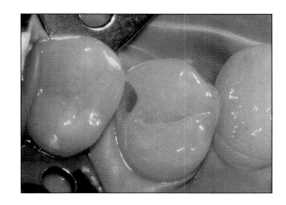

Fig 5-19 Saucer-shaped preparation.

with the insufficient etching pattern in the enamel at the inner side of the tunnel (Fig 5-18). If the adhesive tunnel restorations (Vitremer/Z-100) were directly compared with Ketac Silver restorations, they were superior. One could hypothesize that the results of the polyalkenoate cement could be improved by closing the access cavity with resin composite placed according to adhesive techniques. However, an in vivo study did not show significant effects of such a procedure.[60]

The results of the groups restored with Ariston pHc were completely insufficient. Two reasons might explain this result: (1) the Ariston liner used has poor adhesive properties, and (2) more likely, the extremely high hygroscopic expansion of the material is to blame.[61] Even despite the small (volume) restorations performed in this study, the hygroscopic expansion must have created some enamel cracks in the proximal ridge, which were clearly seen at the occlusal surface in some samples.

The restoration of tunnel cavities with adhesive techniques is a step in the right direction of a minimally invasive approach and offers many advantages, because

(1) by placing the tunnel cavity in the area of the proximal ridge, the distance to the pulp is increased and (2) by locating the preparation in the area of the DEJ, caries excavation is simplified and probably more effective. The risk with these advantages is the greater possibility for a ridge fracture, which can be easily repaired.

Additionally, ozone could be applied to further reduce or totally eliminate the bacteria, if modified applicators were available.

Restorations with external access to a carious lesion

"Saucer-shaped" cavities (Fig 5-19) seem to be ideal for initial minimally invasive intervention, and they show clinically excellent long-term results.[62] However, one must remember that the close relationship to the adjacent teeth presents a high risk for tooth injury, unless space is generated by the use of separating rubber bands.[39]

Cavity design. There is a need to know which design for small proximal cavities yields the best results. In looking at this problem, one must be open to new designs. The cavity shape with thin and un-

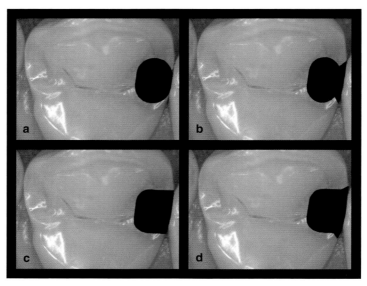

Fig 5-20 The four possible cavity shapes used in the experiment: *(a)* undermined enamel; *(b)* adhesive preparation; *(c)* preparation without bevel; *(d)* preparation with bevel.

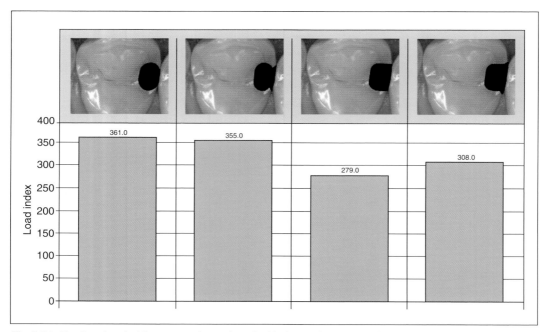

Fig 5-21 Fracture load of the restorations placed with the cavity shapes shown in Fig 5-20.

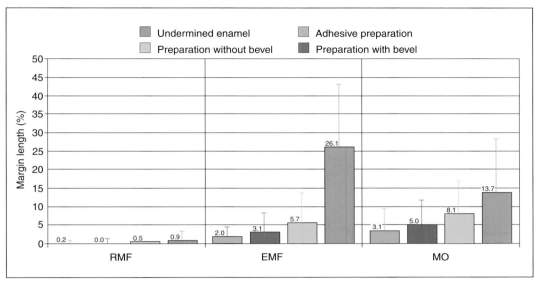

Fig 5-22 Margin quality of the restorations placed with the cavity shapes shown in Fig 5-20. (RMF = restoration margin fracture; EMF = enamel margin fracture; MO = marginal opening.)

dermined enamel tips (Fig 5-20, top left) seems questionable. However, a study has shown that restorations with cervical finishing lines with an inverted bevel showed less dye penetration than restorations prepared with a butt-joint finishing line.[63]

The following experiment was intended to determine the best cavity design for small proximal restorations (Lösche, GM , unpublished data, 2002). In 40 extracted premolars, after initial, coarse cavity preparation, the margins were prepared in the modification shown in Fig 5-20. All cavities were restored with Optibond FL (SDS Kerr, Orange, CA) and Z-100 (3M ESPE). After being subjected to thermocycling (2,000 cycles, 5°C to 55°C), they were stressed with a cyclical load (as described above) until failure. Based on replicas, margin analyses be-

fore and after thermocycling were also performed.

As can be seen in Fig 5-21, there were no significant differences in the fracture fatigue load, although groups with internal retention (ie, adhesive preparation and undermined enamel) performed slightly better.

The results of the margin analysis after thermocycling (Fig 5-22) clearly showed that the restorations with undermined enamel margins had a significantly poorer margin quality than the three other groups. The groups with bevel (adhesive preparation and preparation with bevel) showed better marginal integrity than small box-shaped proximal cavities without bevel. Bevels or long bevels are the best way to guarantee tight restorations in saucer-shaped or small box-shaped proximal cavities.

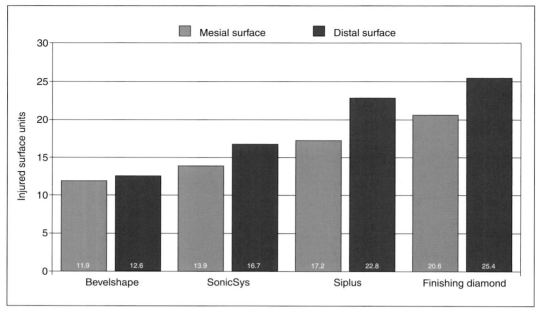

Fig 5-23 The frequency of injuries to adjacent teeth. From Hahn et al.[68] Used with permission.

Methods for cavity preparations. To minimize the danger of injuring adjacent teeth during the preparation of proximal cavities, special preparation methods and instruments were developed.[64–67] Each injured surface unit measured 0.14 mm^2. In evaluating the frequency of injuries (Fig 5-23), Bevelshape files (Intensiv, Viganello Lugano, Switzerland) and SonicSys tips (KaVo) caused fewer injuries than did the Siplus System (Brasseler, Lemgo, Germany) and conventional rotating diamond burs.[68] As a rule, injuries to the tooth surface with the new instruments are not as deep as those occurring with rotating instruments (Fig 5-24).

In a study by Schünemann et al, the effect of different instruments used for beveling the enamel on the margin quality was investigated. The following instruments were used (Fig 5-25):

- 40-μm Bevelshape files
- 46-μm SonicSys microtips
- 15- and 40-μm conventional diamond burs (Composhape, Intensiv)

The margin quality of the composite restorations was investigated in the scanning electron microscope (SEM) at 200× magnification. The results after thermocycling (2000 cycles, 5°C to 55°C) (Fig 5-26) showed that enamel margins finished with the 15-μm rotating diamonds, which were intended as a control group, were as bad as those finished with the Bevelshape files

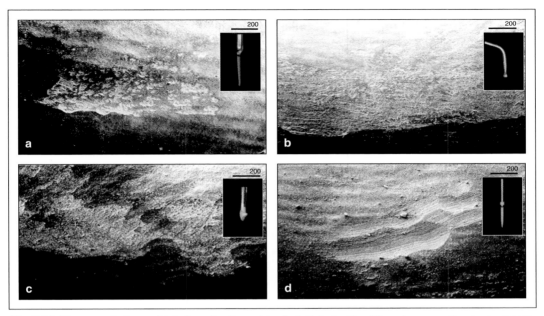

Fig 5-24 The morphology of injuries of adjacent teeth inflicted with different preparation instruments. From Hahn et al.[68] Used with permission.

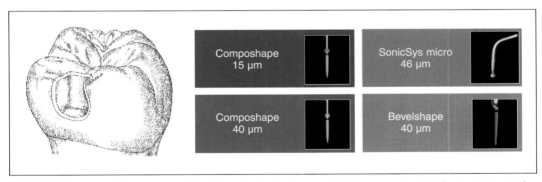

Fig 5-25 Experimental groups used to determine the influence of different preparation instruments on the margin quality. (Based on data from Schünemann et al.[69])

in regard to restoration margin fractures and marginal openings. Furthermore, Bevelshape files created a high number of enamel margin fractures, which can be attributed to the axial movement: This movement creates a loosening of the enamel prisms and causes subsequent microfractures in the cervical enamel.[69]

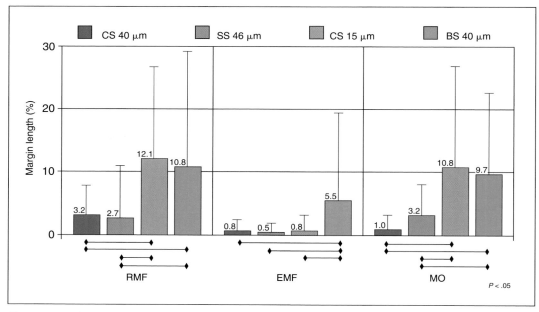

Fig 5-26 Margin quality of the restorations after thermocycling. (CS = Composhape; SS = SonicSys; BS = Bevelshape; RMF = restoration margin fracture; EMF = enamel margin fracture; MO = marginal opening). (Based on data from Schünemann et al.[69])

Access to the lesion and restorative technique. There is a large discrepancy in the performance of composites in in vitro tests and in vivo observations. Ferracane attributes this to handling problems.[70] Therefore, it is reasonable to look at the performance of minimally invasive restorations, including the preparation techniques, the application of the material, and the finishing/polishing of the restoration with an in vitro simulation of the in vivo conditions. The reason to do this is that in vivo, because of their location, the margins to be assessed are difficult to access for investigation. Furthermore, the simulation procedure has the advantage that afterward the restorations can be submitted to standardized stress in the laboratory. An additional advantage is that the restoration may be finished and polished under ideal conditions and thus may be evaluated without artifacts that are created during finishing and polishing under adverse conditions in vivo.

The question of which cavity design and which access is the best for a minimally invasive procedure in the proximal area of posterior teeth is still unanswered. Therefore, an experiment was designed to answer this question. In a simulation model, three experienced

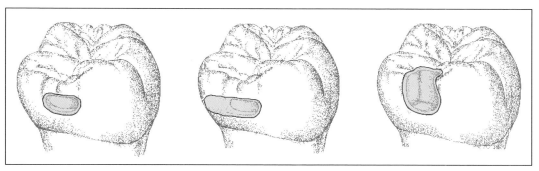

Fig 5-27 In vivo simulation of the placement of minimally invasive restorations with different access cavities.

dentists were required to place a total of 15 restorations, 5 restorations each with a direct, lateral, or occlusal approach for a small proximal lesion in posterior teeth using conventional rotating diamond burs and the SonicSys Micro System (Fig 5-27). The direct approach yields a one-surface restoration, which is only possible if clinically the adjacent tooth is prepared for a restoration, thus allowing direct access to the lesion. The lateral access was described by Battock et al to restore proximal root-caries lesions.[71] Since the introduction of oscillating preparation instruments working in the sonic or ultrasonic range, this access is also possible in close proximity of the contact point. The third group was the control, using very conservative Class 2 cavity preparations. The cavities were restored using the total-etch technique with Optibond FL (SDS Kerr) and Tetric Flow (Ivoclar Vivadent) for the cavities with direct or lateral access and Tetric Ceram (Ivoclar Vivadent) for the cavities with occlusal access (Class 2). The restorations were finished and polished in situ. Proximal overhangs were removed with scalpel blades first (BB 512, Aesculap, Tuttlingen, Germany). Further finishing and polishing were done with aluminum oxide–coated strips (Soflex, 3M ESPE).

The teeth with the polished restorations were removed from the models and subjected to thermocycling (2000 cycles, 5°C to 55°C). After replicas were made with a polyvinyl siloxane impression material, the restorations were recontoured, finished, and polished under visual control. Then replicas were made again for further SEM evaluation. Figure 5-28 shows the evaluation of the margin areas marked in red in the SEM at 200× magnification. The distribution of areas rated "excellent margin" and "marginal irregularity" was almost identical. Overhangs and marginal openings were found more often in restorations placed with lateral access. Refinishing under visual control was able to eliminate all overhangs. Fur-

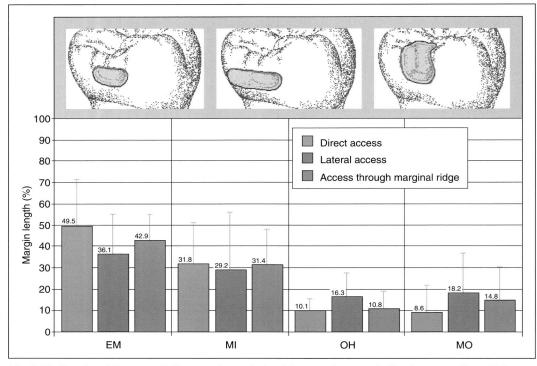

Fig 5-28 Results of the quantitative margin analysis of the margins in red after thermocycling. (EM = excellent margin; MI = marginal imperfections; OH = overhangs; MO = marginal opening).

thermore, the amount of marginal openings was also reduced (Fig 5-29); it can therefore be interpreted that poorly adapted and overcontoured margins lead to misinterpretations. As seen after thermocycling, also after recontouring/refinishing/repolishing, restorations placed with lateral access showed a higher amount of marginal openings in the area right below the contact point. The explanation for this pattern is evident in Fig 5-30. Because of the close contact with the adjacent tooth and semispherical shape of the SonicSys instrument, the resulting cavity shape has a butt-joint finishing line instead of a bevel. Thus, as shown above, these are inferior conditions for a reliable

adhesive bond of the composite. Therefore, it can be concluded that also for cavities with a lateral access, the separation of the teeth with rubber bands prior to intervention is beneficial because it allows an optimal finishing line for bonding. In a subsequent investigation cone-shaped SonicSys instruments were used in the above-mentioned indication with full satisfaction (Lösche GM, unpublished data, 2000).

Conclusions

Few things have changed dentistry more than the profound knowledge about

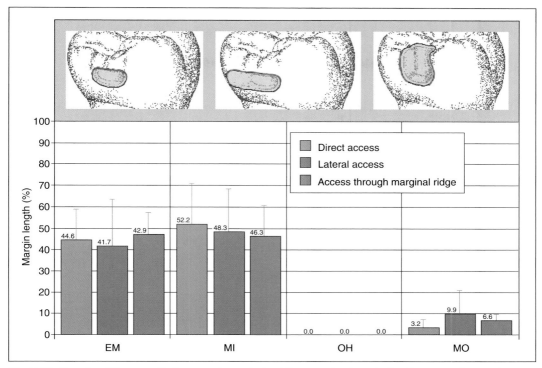

Fig 5-29 Results of the quantitative margin analysis of the margins in red after thermocycling and recontouring/finishing/polishing under visual control. (EM = excellent margin; MI = marginal imperfections; OH = overhangs; MO = marginal opening).

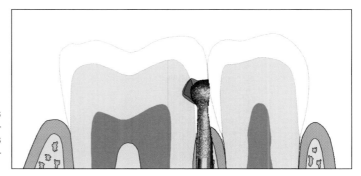

Fig 5-30 If a SonicSys microtip is used in close proximity to the contact point with lateral access, its function is limited and yields a butt-joint finishing line.

caries and the use of adhesive technology. For a long time the role of the restorative dentist was very limited. Clinicians just waited until a carious lesion had developed into a marked cavity before they removed the decayed tissue and replaced it with a restorative material. Today, responsible minimally invasive operative dentistry consists of the following:

- Early diagnosis, classification, and monitoring of carious lesions
- Evaluation of the individual caries risk factors
- Reduction of the pathogenic and cariogenic flora to prevent the growth of carious lesions
- Remineralization and monitoring of initial lesions with an intact surface
- Restoration of cavities with minimally invasive cavity preparations and the best possible adhesive techniques

References

1. Splieth C, Förster M, Meyer G. Vergleich der Lokalfluoridierung und Fissurenversiegelung zur Kariesprophylaxe an ersten permanenten Molaren bei Kindern. Dtsch Zahnärztl Z 1998; 53:799–804.

2. Irmisch B. Kariesprophylaxe mittels Fissurenversiegelung. Dtsch Zahnärtl Z 1992;47:790–796.

3. Llodra JC, Bravo M, Delgado Rodriguez M, et al. Factors influencing the effectiveness of sealants—A meta-analysis. Community Dent Oral Epidemiol 1993;21:261–218.

4. Simonsen RJ. Retention and effectiveness of dental sealant after 15 years. J Am Dent Assoc 1991;122:34–42.

5. Wagner M, Lutz F, Menghini GD, et al. Erfahrungsbericht über Fissruenversiegelungen in der Privatpraxis mit einer Liegedauer bis zu zehn Jahren. Schweiz Monatsschr Zahnmed 1994;104:156–159.

6. Chosack A, Eidelman E. Effect of the time from application until exposure to light on the tag lengths of a visible light–polymerized sealant. Dent Mater 1988;4:302–306.

7. Mertz Fairhurst EJ, Curtis JW Jr, Ergle JW, et al. Ultraconservative and cariostatic sealed restorations: Results at year 10. J Am Dent Assoc 1998;129:55–66.

8. Lussi A, Firestone A, Schoenberg V, et al. In vivo diagnosis of fissure caries using a new electrical resistance monitor. Caries Res 1995;29:81–87.

9. Lussi A, Imwinkelried S, Pitts N, et al. Performance and reproducibility of a laser fluorescence system for detection of occlusal caries in vitro. Caries Res 1999;33:261–266.

10. Holmes J, Lynch E. Reversal of occlusal caries using air abrasion, ozone and sealing [abstract 3468]. J Dent Res 2004;82:403.

11. Lussi A. Methoden zur Diagnose und Verlaufsdiagnose der Karies. Wann bohren? Dtsch Zahnärztl Z 1998;53:175–182.

12. Bille J, Thylstrup A. Radiographic diagnosis and clinical tissue changes in relation to treatment of approximal carious lesions. Caries Res 1982; 16:1–6.

13. Lunder N, von der Fehr FR. Approximal cavitation related to bite-wing image and caries activity in adolescents. Caries Res 1996;30:143–147.

14. Rimmer PA, Pitts NB. Temporary elective tooth separation as a diagnostic aid in general dental practice. Br Dent J 1990;169:87–92.

15. Rugg-Gunn AJ. Approximal carious lesion. A comparison of the radiological and clinical appearance. Br Dent J 1972;133:481–484.

16. Pitts NB, Renson CE. Image analysis of bitewing radiographs: A histologically validated comparison with visual assessments of radiolucency depth in enamel. Br Dent J 1986;160:205–209.

17. Mayer R. Ästhetisch-adhäsive Füllungstherapie im Seitenzahngebiet—eine Illusion? Dtsch Zahnärztl Z 1991;46:468–470.

18. Lösche GM, Hilbig WH, Roulet J-F. The margin quality of direct posterior composite restorations close to the CEJ [abstract 1889]. J Dent Res 1992:752.

19. Lösche GM. Marginal adaptation of Class II composite fillings: Guided polymerization vs reduced light intensity. J Adhes Dent 1999;1:31–9.

20. Haak R, Lösche GM, Roulet J-F. Bond strength of composite resin to cervical enamel and dentin [abstract 190]. J Dent Res 1996;75:41.

21. Pfeiffer P, Schmage P, Nergiz I, et al. Effects of different exposure values on diagnostic accuracy of digital images. Quintessence Int 2000; 31:257–260.

22. Wenzel A, Borg E, Hintze H, et al. Accuracy of caries diagnosis in digital images from charge-coupled device and storage phosphor systems: An in vitro study. Dentomaxillofac Radiol 1995;24:250–254.

23. Gröndahl HG. Radiographic assessment of caries and caries progression. In: Anusavice KJ (ed). Quality Evaluation of Dental Restorations: Criteria for Placement and Replacement. Chicago: Quintessence 1989:151–167.

24. Bader JD, Shugars DA. Agreement among dentists' recommendations for restorative treatment. J Dent Res 1993;72:891–896.

25. Kay EJ, Knill Jones R. Variation in restorative treatment decisions: Application of Receiver Operating Characteristic curve (ROC) analysis. Community Dent Oral Epidemiol 1992;20:113–117.

26. Kay EJ, Nuttall NM. Relationship between dentists' treatment attitudes and restorative decisions made on the basis of simulated bitewing radiographs. Community Dent Oral Epidemiol 1994;22:71–74.

27. Swan ES, Lewis DW. Ontario dentists: 2. Bitewing utilization and restorative treatment decisions. J Can Dent Assoc 1993;59:68–70.

28. Mileman PA, Mulder E, Van der Weele L. Factors influencing the likelihood of successful decisions to treat dentin caries from bitewing radiographs. Community Dent Oral Epidemiol 1992;20:175–180.

29. Noar SJ, Smith BG. Diagnosis of caries and treatment decisions in approximal surfaces of posterior teeth in vitro. J Oral Rehabil 1990;17:209–218.

30. Heaven TJ, Firestone AR, Feagin FF. Computer-aided image analysis of natural approximal caries on radiographic films. J Dent Res 1991;71:846–849.

31. Heaven TJ, Firestone AR, Feagin FF. Quantitative radiographic measurement of dentinal lesions. J Dent Res 1990;69:51–54.

32. Pitts NB, Renson CE. Reproducibility of computer-aided image-analysis-derived estimates of the depth and area of radiolucencies in approximal enamel. J Dent Res 1985;64:1221–1224.

33. Duncan RC, Heaven T, Weems RA, et al. Using computers to diagnose and plan treatment of approximal caries. Detected in radiographs. J Am Dent Assoc 1995;126:873–882.

34. Shrout MK, Russell CM, Potter BJ, et al. Spatial resolution in radiometric analysis of enamel loss. A pilot study. Oral Surg Oral Med Oral Pathol Oral Radiol Endod 1996;81:245–250.

35. Thylstrup A, Bille J, Qvist V. Radiographic and observed tissue changes in approximal carious lesions at the time of operative treatment. Caries Res 1986;20:75–85.

36. Hintze H, Wenze A. Clinical and laboratory radiographic caries diagnosis. A study of the same teeth. Dentomaxillofac Radiol 1996;25:115–118.

37. Kogon SL, Stephens RG, Reid JA, et al. Can radiographic criteria be used to distinguish between cavitated and noncavitated approximal enamel caries? Dentomaxillofac Radiol 1987;16:33–36.

38. Stokes AN. Elastomeric separation to aid the diagnosis and treatment of anterior proximal caries lesions. N Z Dent J 1989;85:90–92.

39. Bjarnason S. Temporary tooth separation in the treatment of approximal carious lesions. Quintessence Int 1996;27:249–251.

40. Ratledge DK, Kidd EA, Beighton D. A clinical and microbiological study of approximal carious lesions. Part 2: Efficacy of caries removal following tunnel and Class II cavity preparations. Caries Res 2001;35:8–11.

41. Mount GJ, Ngo H. Minimal intervention: Early lesions. Quintessence Int 2000;31:535–546.

42. Sedden RP. The detection of cavitation in carious approximal surfaces in vivo by tooth separation, impression and scanning electron microscopy. J Dent 1989;17:117–120.

43. Longbottom C, Huysmans MC, Pitts NB, et al. Detection of dental decay and its extent using a.c. impedance spectroscopy. Nat Med 1996;2:235–237.

44. Huysmans MC, Longbottom C, Pitts NB, et al. Impedance spectroscopy of teeth with and without approximal caries lesions—an in vitro study. J Dent Res 1996;75:1871-1878.

45. Medeiros VA, Seddon RP. Iatrogenic damage to approximal surfaces in contact with Class II restorations. J Dent 2000;28:103–110.

46. Strübing W, Opitz J. Präparationsdefekte an Nachbarzähnen bei Inlay- und Kronenversorgungen. Dtsch Zahnärztl Z 2000;55:101–113.

47. Lussi A. Verletzung der Nachbarzähne bei der Präparation approximaler Kavitäten. Schweiz Monatsschr Zahnmed 1995;105:1259–1264.

48. Tyas MJ, Anusavice KJ, Frencken JE, Mount GJ. Minimal intervention dentistry: A review. FDI Commission Project 1–97. Int Dent J 2000; 50:1–12.

49. Strand GV, Tveit AB, Gjerdet NR, et al. Marginal ridge strength of teeth with tunnel preparations. Int Dent J 1995;45:117–123.

50. Strand GV, Tveit AB. Effectiveness of caries removal by the partial tunnel preparation method. Scand J Dent Res 1993;101:270–273.

51. Strand GV, Tveit AB, Espelid I. Variations among operators in the performance of tunnel preparations in vitro. Scand J Dent Res 1994;102: 151–155.

52. Strand GV, Tveit AB, Eide GE. Cavity design and dimensions of tunnel preparations versus composite resin Class II preparations. Acta Odontol Scand 1995;53:217–221.

53. Strand GV, Nordbo H, Leirskar J, et al. Tunnel restorations placed in routine practice and observed for 24 to 54 months. Quintessence Int 2000;31:453–460.

54. Hasselrot L. Tunnel restorations in permanent teeth. A 7-year follow-up study. Swed Dent J 1998;22:1–7.

55. Holst A, Brännstrom M. Restoration of small proximal dentin lesions with the tunnel technique. A 3-year clinical study performed in Public Dental Service clinics. Swed Dent J 1998;22: 143–148.

56. Papa J, Cain C, Messer HH. Efficacy of tunnel restorations in the removal of caries. Quintessence Int 1993;24:715–719.

57. Preston AJ, Higham SM, Agalamanyi EA, Mair LH. Fluoride recharge of aesthetic dental materials. J Oral Rehabil 1999;26:936-940.

58. Pereira AC, Basting RT, Pinelli C, De Castro Meneghim M, Werner CW. Retention and caries preventin of Vitremer and Ketac-Bond used as occlusal sealants. Am J Dent 1999;12: 62-64.

59. Creanor SL, Awawdeh LA, Saunders WP, Foye RH, Gilmour WH. The effect of a resin-modified glass ionomer restorative material on artificially demineralised dentine caries in vitro. J Dent 1998;26:527-531.

60. Pilebro CE, van Dijken JW, Stenberg R. Durability of tunnel restorations in general practice: A 3-year multicenter study. Acta Odontol Scand 1999;57:35–39.

61. Martin N, Jedynakiewicz NM, Fisher AC. Hygroscopic expansion and solubility of composite restoratives. Dent Mater 2003;19:77–86.

62. Nordbo H, Leirskar J, von der Fehr FR. Saucer-shaped cavity preparations for posterior approximal resin composite restorations: Observations up to 10 years. Quintessence Int 1998;29:5–11.

63. Holan G, Eidelman E, Wright GZ. The effect of internal bevel on marginal leakage at the approximal surface of Class 2 composite restorations. Oper Dent 1997;22:217–221.

64. Hugo B. Neue Präparations—Restaurationsmethoden zur defektbezogenen Versorgung approximaler Karies (1). Quintessenz Zahnärztl Lit 1996;47:911–923.

65. Hugo B. Neue Präparations—Restaurationsmethoden zur defektbezogenen Versorgung approximaler Karies (II). Quintess Zahnärztl Lit 1996;47:1051–1069.

66. Krejci I, Dietschi D, Lutz FU. Principles of proximal cavity preparation and finishing with ultrasonic diamond tips. Pract Periodontics Aesthet Dent 1998;10:295–298.

67. Lussi A, Gygax M. Präparationstechnik zur signifikanten Minimierung von Nachbarzahnverletzungen. Acta Med Dent Helv 1996;1:3–6.

68. Hahn P, Günther F, Hellwig E. Einfluß verschiedener Präparationstechniken auf die Verletzung von Nachbarzähnen und die Qualität der Schmelzabschrägung. Dtsch Zahnärztl Z 2000;55:118–123.

69. Schünemann TH, Lösche GM, Roulet J-F. The influence of preparation systems on marginal adaptation of Class II fillings [abstract 389]. J Dent Res 1998;77:680.

70. Ferracane JL. Using posterior composites appropriately. J Am Dent Assoc 1992;123:53-58.

71. Battock RD, Rhoades J, Lund MR. Management of proximal caries on the roots of posterior teeth. Oper Dent 1979;4:108–112.

Chapter 6

Materials for Minimally Invasive Treatments

Marc Braem

Abstract

Materials for minimally invasive treatments should be able to withstand the same masticatory forces exerted on their occlusal contact surfaces as do materials selected for large cavities. Due to cavity geometry, in the case of adhesive bonding of a small restoration, one can expect increased internal stresses, at least when there is insufficient or no flow compensation.

The results of in vitro tests of Young's modulus and fatigue limits of various restorative materials show that, in view of the physiological stresses, a more rapid fatigue failure is likely to occur within the group of conventional glass-ionomer restoratives. With the help of scanning electron microscopy, the fracture surfaces also reveal that the manipulation of the material by the clinician often yields to internal defects that will render the restoration more prone to fatigue failure. This chapter discusses the stresses that occur in restorative materials at the surface and subsurface levels following occlusal contacts and thereby focuses on crack-growth phenomena. Since crack growth is suspected of playing a role in wear processes, it is of primary importance in the understanding of damage accumulation in restorative materials.

The concept of minimal intervention dentistry has evolved from a better understanding of caries progression.[1] It is recommended to remove only the infected tooth structure, thus saving the maximum amount of sound tooth tissue. Although the preservation of tooth structure has always been the primary goal in operative dentistry, the advent of adhesive materials has created the opportunity to divert from an architectural cavity shape toward an outline as dictated by the lesion.

The cavity size will range from infinitely small to several millimeters. The restorative materials to be used will have to comply with several requirements.[2] They should bond to both enamel and dentin to seal the cavity and possess bioactive properties such as fluoride release, antimicrobial properties, and remineralization capacity, as well as mechanical and physical properties that promote appropriate handling characteristics and adequate resistance against deformation and loading. The restorative materials should also promote biomimetics.

This chapter will focus on the properties of contemporary restorative materials that, when subjected to cyclic loading, comply with the specific requirements for minimal intervention treatment.

Table 6-1 Materials tested

Material	Shade	Batch	Manufacturer
Silux Plus	U	0AM2-92LO8A	3M, St Paul, MN
Z100	A2	Lot 92D14A	3M, St Paul, MN
Z100 Single-Dose Capsule	UD	19960410	3M, St Paul, MN
P50-APC	U	Lot E8JD03	3M, St Paul, MN
Vitremer	A4	P: 199-30-405 L: 199-31-218	3M, St Paul, MN
F2000	A3	Lot 19970828	3M, St Paul, MN
Filtek P60	A3	19990318	3M, St Paul, MN
Filtek Z250	A3	19990519	3M, St Paul, MN
Tetric Ceram	A3	922793	Ivoclar Vivadent, Schaan, Liechtenstein
Ariston pHc	Clear	B02922	Ivoclar Vivadent, Schaan, Liechtenstein

P = powder
L = liquid

(continued)

Study Design

Materials

The materials used in the study were selected to represent a wide cross-section of material types having widely different composition and properties. Some older products were included for reason of comparison (Table 6-1).

Rectangular samples were made in Plexiglass molds covered with a thin layer of Vaseline. Light-cured materials were polymerized for 3 minutes in a modified light oven (Unilux AC, Heraeus Kulzer, Wehrheim, Germany) operating with visible light of 450 to 520 nm and with absolute time intervals. The proportions in powder-liquid formulations were respected by weighing (Mettler Instrumente, Type College 244, Greifensee-Zurich, Switzerland) the respective amounts. Indirect composites were prepared using the appropriate equipment following the instructions of the manufacturers. All samples were machined to their final dimensions (length = 35 mm, depth = 1.2 mm, width = 5 mm). Samples were stored in distilled water at 37°C for 1 month (WTB Binder APT Line BED53, Tuttlingen, Germany) prior to testing under humid conditions.

Table 6-1 (continued) Materials tested

Material	Shade	Batch	Manufacturer
Targis Dentin	210	Lot 15553	Ivoclar Vivadent, Schaan, Liechtenstein
Charisma	OA22	22	Heraeus Kulzer, Wehrheim, Germany
Solitaire II	A2	VP190399/Ju	Heraeus Kulzer, Wehrheim, Germany
Herculite XRV	U	jan/93	Kerr, Romulus, MN
Prodigy Condensable	A2	904665	Kerr, Orange, CA
belleGlass HP	A3	Lot 909D89	Kerr, Orange, CA
HiFi Master Palette	A3.5	P: BN069428-4 L: BN039430-1	Shofu, Tonbridge, UK
Shofu Type II	#1 universal shade	P: 189401 L: 629412	Shofu, Tonbridge, UK
Shofu FX	universal	P: 019605 L: 729604	Shofu, Tonbridge, UK
Pertac II	A3	006 34764	ESPE, Seefeld, Germany
Sinfony	DA3	Lot FW0056688	ESPE, Seefeld, Germany
Fuji II LC capsules	B3	Lot 121-045 Lot 021-231	GC, Tokyo, Japan
Fuji II LC powder-liquid	B3	P: lot 160-931 L: lot 240-831	GC, Tokyo, Japan
Fuji IX GP capsules	A2	Lot 020967	GC, Tokyo, Japan
Gradia	DA3	9910261	GC, Tokyo, Japan
Dyract	A2	Lot 94-05-20-Z	De Trey/Dentsply, Konstanz, Germany
Surefil	A	980902	Dentsply/Caulk, Milford, DE
Admira	A2	93536	Voco, Cuxhaven, Germany
Alert	A2	21229	Jeneric/Pentron, Wallingford, CT
Glacier	A3	990322	SDI, Victoria, Australia
Pyramid Dentin	A1	9900005548	Bisco, Schaumburg, IL
Quadrant Posterior Dense	A2	VP190399ju	Cavex Holland BV, Haarlem, Holland
Synergy Compact	A2/B2	IF674	Coltène/Whaledent, Altstätten, Switzerland

Young's Modulus and Fatigue Resistance

The testing device and procedure have been described in detail[3] and are discussed here only schematically. Two electromagnets mounted in opposing directions were used to produce an adjustable load. Since this load is reversed for reasons of dynamic creep compensation, the samples were clamped between two opposite supports. This situation is referred to as *clamped*. Load control was established using two piezoelectric force transducers (Kistler 9205, Kistler, Winterthur, Switzerland) on top of each shaft. The force transducers were connected to a measuring unit (Kistler 5011) and controlled by computer via a data acquisition board (AT-MIO-16H-9, National Instruments, Zaventem, Belgium). A frictionless deflection meter (LVDT Roltran E. Schaevitz, Type 200HR, Brussels, Belgium) coupled to a measuring unit (Kistler 5851 AY27) monitored the bending of the test samples and was controlled by the computer. The machine can be used in a quasistatic way to determine the Young's modulus in a three-point bending configuration.

Assuming three periods of 15 minutes of chewing per day at a chewing rate of 1 Hz, the number of chews is 2,700 per day.[4] This adds up to about 1×10^6 times per year. At this frequency, a fatigue test on one sample takes about 12 days to accomplish. Increasing the rate to 2 Hz offers a time-saving approach well within the frequency dependency range of the tested viscoelastic materials. If the noncontact events are eliminated from the chewing cycles, 10,000 cycles represents about 1.2 months of real-life contact.

The flexural fatigue limit (FFL) was determined according to the "staircase" method, as a function of the clamped fracture strength and a given number of cycles. If the sample did not fail within 10,000 cycles, the stress level for the next test sample was increased by a fixed amount. If failure did occur, the stress level for the next sample was accordingly decreased. Based on the number of failures and nonfailures, both linked to the tested stress level, the FFL can be statistically calculated. The result is a stress level (in megapascals) at which 50% of the tested samples will survive.

Scanning Electron Microscopic Fractography

Fractured surfaces were used for investigation with a scanning electron microscope (SEM). They were mounted on aluminum stubs and gold plated (Sputtering device 07 120, Balzers Union, Balzers, Liechtenstein), and studied thereafter in the SEM.

Results

Table 6-2 shows the results for the Young's modulus and FFL after 1 month of water sorption at 37°C. The results from both tests indicate a wide variety in resistance against deformation.

The Young's modulus of the conventional glass-ionomer cements could not be measured because of their brittle nature. The results indicate that the Young's modulus of a given category of resin composite materials, such as packable composites, is not as homogeneous as might be expected. The resin-modified

Table 6-2 Results for Young's modulus (E) and flexural fatigue limit (FFL) for the tested materials after 1 month of water sorption

Material	E (GPa ± SD)	FFL (MPa ± SD)
Microfilled composites		
Silux Plus	7.7 ± 0.3	54.6 ± 3.4
Artglass	8.0 ± 0.4	77.8 ± 2.7
Hybrid composites		
Charisma	11.5 ± 2.1	60.1 ± 3.0
P50 APC	19.1 ± 1.3	74.9 ± 3.6
Z100	16.7 ± 0.7	94.5 ± 3.7
Z100 Single-Dose Capsules	16.1 ± 0.4	78.2 ± 3.6
Filtek Z250	12.2 ± 0.4	75.8 ± 2.7
Herculite XRV	16.7 ± 0.1	112.0 ± 15.9
Pertac II	12.9 ± 0.7	113.9 ± 9.8
Packable/condensable/ moldable composites		
Ariston AT*	10.6 ± 0.8	58.1 ± 3.6
SureFil*	15.5 ± 0.8	79.4 ± 5.3
Alert*	18.4 ± 0.3	69.8 ± 5.3
Pyramid Dentin*	15.5 ± 0.3	60.9 ± 12.0
Prodigy Condensable*	14.5 ± 0.4	54.4 ± 7.3
Synergy Compact*	13.6 ± 0.6	59.2 ± 5.6
Glacier*	12.8 ± 0.4	53.9 ± 4.3
Solitaire II*	12.6 ± 0.4	38.0 ± 1.7
Quadrant Posterior Dense*	12.4 ± 0.8	40.5 ± 1.3
Tetric Ceram	9.2 ± 0.5	64.6 ± 3.7
Filtek P60	11.8 ± 0.4	68.9 ± 4.2
Indirect composites		
Gradia	7.6 ± 0.8	61.7 ± 1.9
Targis	7.6 ± 0.8	76.5 ± 4.1
belleGlass HP	20.0 ± 0.9	89.7 ± 8.2
Sinfony	4.7 ± 0.2	48.9 ± 2.2

Table 6-2 (continued) Results for Young's modulus (E) and flexural fatigue limit (FFL) for the tested materials after 1 month of water sorption

Material	E (GPa ± SD)	FFL (MPa ± SD)
Conventional glass ionomers		
HiFi Master Palette[†]	—	35.2 ± 3.0
Shofu Type II[†]	—	26.9 ± 1.6
Shofu FX[†]	—	28.8 ± 4.6
Fuji IX GP capsules[†]	—	27.3 ± 2.4
Resin-modified glass ionomers		
Vitremer	10.2 ± 1.0	53.2 ± 2.0
Fuji II LC capsules	8.6 ± 0.4	51.0 ± 3.5
Fuji II LC powder-liquid	8.6 ± 0.4	51.1 ± 8.2
Polyacid-modified composites		
F2000	20.8 ± 1.3	58.4 ± 4.3
Dyract	11.6 ± 0.4	67.2 ± 5.1

*Data taken from Abe and coworkers[5,6]
[†]It was not possible to measure the Young's modulus because the samples failed during the testing procedure.

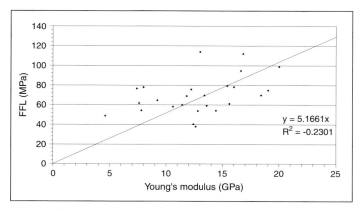

Fig 6-1 Regression analysis showed no correlation between the Young's modulus and FFL.

glass-ionomer cements show a resistance against deformation that is comparable with at least that of the microfilled composites. The polyacid modified materials tested are comparable to the hybrid materials as far as the Young's modulus is concerned.

As for the fatigue resistance, it is difficult to attribute a general fatigue behavior to a category of materials, especially the composite materials. The resin-modified glass ionomers, however, show comparable results within their group.

From the present findings, it is further obvious that the ranking of the materials according to the Young's modulus is not necessarily identical to the ranking based on the fatigue resistance. This is further confirmed by regression analysis between both properties (Fig 6-1) that reveals a lack of correlation.

Clinical Implications

The Young's modulus of resin composites is dictated more by the structure of the material than by a classification relying on vague properties such as "packable."[7] This is again revealed in the present study, where a regression analysis of the Young's modulus of the tested materials versus the volumetric filler fraction yields a high correlation coefficient ($R^2 = 0.98$), as is reported in the literature. This being true, it does not, however, allow for the selection of almost any of the tested materials to replace lost dental tissue. Indeed, if a clinical situation requires that a replacement material possess a Young's modulus of at least that of dentin, around 18 GPa, almost none of the materials tested would fulfill this criterion. On the other hand, at present there is no evidence from clinical studies that materials with a Young's modulus of less than 18 GPa would systematically fail during service. So, although the Young's modulus reveals substantial information for the resistance against deformation, by itself this property will not allow for the proper selection of a material from the list.

The variation in the results for the FFL of the composites is different from that of the quasistatic Young's modulus. Furthermore, the property of fatigue resistance is not reflected in the volumetric filler fraction of the materials: A regression analysis reveals only a very weak correlation ($R^2 = 0.32$). This could indicate that the fatigue resistance is linked with all the different phases a material is built upon and on the way these phases interact. To further evaluate this interaction, the fracture surfaces of some of the materials for which the filler and matrix phase are physically distinct phases, such as composites, were studied using SEM.

The SEM fractography reveals that the crack runs along the interface area between organic filler particles and matrix phase, as shown in Fig 6-2. Further analysis should point out whether the failure is adhesive or cohesive in nature. The loss of interaction between filler phase and matrix phase was found to be the most dominant failure pattern in composites as well as in polyacid modified composites (Fig 6-3). These findings reveal the importance of a good coupling phase

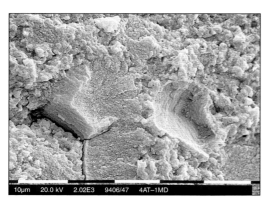

Fig 6-2 Scanning electron microscopic view of Gradia showing the failure along the interface between the large organic filler particles and the matrix phase. (Original magnification ×2,000.)

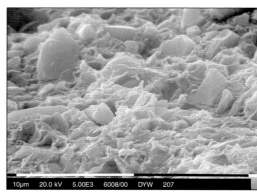

Fig 6-3 Scanning electron microscopic view of Dyract. Several particles can be observed that are no longer coupled to the matrix phase, following failure after fatigue. (Original magnification ×5,000.)

and illustrate the possible detrimental effects of contamination during the pretreatment of silanization of composite fillers.[8] With this in mind, and without knowing the effect of fatigue on filler-matrix interaction, one could also question the leaching of ions from filler particles in a composite system.

The results for the resin-modified glass-ionomer cements are at the lower end of the composite results. This is a promising finding, especially because of the bioactive properties of these materials with regard to fluoride release. The results are also better in absolute values than those obtained by the conventional glass-ionomer cements.

The question about the minimal requirements for fatigue resistance again arises. There are no data available that describe the fatigue behavior of dentin or enamel. Assuming that functional chewing forces[9] are a magnitude of about 5 to 20 N and assuming that the antagonistic

tooth contact is about 1 mm,[5] the resulting stress in the restoration can account for 5 to 20 MPa. This is well below the FFLs of the studied products, except for the conventional glass-ionomer cements, which had an FFL of about 27 to 35 MPa in humid conditions. This type of restorative material will thus be stressed to its FFL more frequently, especially considering that higher peak stresses often can occur.

References

1. Mount GJ, Ngo H. Minimal intervention: A new concept for operative dentistry. Quintessence Int 2000;31:527–533.

2. Peters MC, McLean ME. Minimal invasive operative care, II. Contemporary techniques and materials: An overview. J Adhes Dent 2001;3:17–31.

3. Braem M, Davidson CL, Lambrechts P, Vanherle G. In vitro flexural fatigue limits of dental composites. J Biomed Mater Res 1994;28:1397–1402.

4. Wiskott HWA, Nicholls JI, Belser UC. Fatigue resistance of soldered joints: A methodological study. Dent Mater 1994;10:215–220.

5. Abe Y, Lambrechts P, Braem MJA, et al. Fatigue behavior of 'packable' composites. Biomaterials (in press).

6. Abe Y, Lambrechts P, Inoue S, et al. Dynamic elastic modulus of 'packable' composites. Dent Mater 2001;17:520–525.

7. Willems G, Lambrechts P, Braem M, Celis JP, Vanherle G. A classification of dental composites according to their morphological and mechanical characteristics. Dent Mater 1992;8: 310–319.

8. Shirai K, Yoshida Y, Nakayama Y, et al. Assessment of decontamination methods as pretreatment of silanization of composite glass fillers. J Biomed Mater Res (Appl Biomater) 2000;53: 204–210.

9. De Boever JA, McCall WD Jr, Holden S, Ash MM Jr. Functional occlusal forces: An investigation by telemetry. J Prosthet Dent 1978;40:326–333.

Chapter 7

Minimally Invasive Dentistry Using Ozone

Aylin Baysan, Edward Lynch

Abstract

Ozone application using the HealOzone system (KaVo, Biberach, Germany) for either 10 or 20 seconds has been proven to dramatically reduce most of the microorganisms in root carious lesions without any adverse effects. Leathery noncavitated primary root caries can easily be arrested nonoperatively with ozone. This treatment regimen is an effective alternative to conventional drilling and filling. No injections, drilling, or filling are required, and the treatment method is exceptionally cost-effective and cost-efficient compared with traditional alternative methods of drilling and filling. Several clinical trials have been completed proving the efficacy of this novel treatment method.

In the United Kingdom, the proportions of people with root-surface restorations rose steadily, with 35% being 55 to 64 years old and 43% being 65 years and older.[1] In 1968, only 21% of people aged 65 to 74 years had any teeth compared with 66% in 1998. Elderly people are now retaining more of their teeth, and the prevalence of root caries increases in the dentate older population. This leads to more complex restorative challenges for clinicians since the treatment of root caries poses a number of problems. Visibility and isolation from oral fluids (saliva, gingival secretion, or hemorrhage) are particular problems, while the maintenance of pulpal integrity through the application of biologically acceptable dressings to the pulp-dentin complex reduces the depth of lesions but does not provide the esthetic, physical, and mechanical qualities required for a restoration. Furthermore, the dental materials available for restoration of primary root caries lesions (PRCLs) include amalgam, resin composite, and glass-ionomer cement, but many problems (ie, microleakage and poor marginal adaptations) have arisen that have necessitated the frequent replacement of restorative materials.[2] While all these materials have their merits, they also have limitations in the restoration of carious lesions in conservative dentistry.

The clinical success of amalgam is well-established when compared with other dental materials for the treatment of root caries. However, amalgam cannot be used in areas where esthetics are of prime importance.[3] Therefore, there is a movement in dentistry toward esthetic restorations. Resin-based composites are now being used as either amalgam substitutes or amalgam alternatives. It should be noted that composites have no caries-preventive effects, and postoperative sensitivity, discoloration, and recurrent caries are often observed in root caries treated with composite.[3] Incorporation of fluoride into resin composite materials has failed to show any beneficial effect in reducing demineralization of root caries lesions when compared with glass-ionomer cements.[4–7] Indeed, secondary caries has been reported as the most common reason for replacement of Class V amalgam, resin composite, or glass-ionomer restorations.[8] Placement of a restoration may result in the tooth being subjected to a repeat restoration cycle in which the restoration may ultimately fail and be replaced by progressively larger restorations.[9]

Glass-ionomer restorative cements are best used for the restoration of erosion and abrasion lesions and PRCLs; however, there are still limitations regarding their tensile strength and low impact and fracture resistance (brittleness).[10] Yip et al[11] reported the surface roughness of eight esthetic restorative materials and relationships with weight changes during fluoride release and uptake. Specimens of various restorative materials were prepared and immersed in 2 mL of artificial saliva at 37°C. The changes in specimen weight and fluoride release were monitored for 12 weeks. This procedure was repeated after recharging the specimens with 1.23% acidulated phosphate fluoride (APF) gel for another 12 weeks. Yip et al[11] reported that there was a significant weight loss for all glass-ionomer cements following APF gel application, which correlated with fluoride release. Mean roughness measurements and scanning electron microscopy showed that the degree of roughness increased from the resin composite to the conventional glass-ionomer cements. It was concluded that the marked erosive effect of APF gel on glass-ionomer restorations could increase surface colonization by plaque microorganisms and reduce the longevity of the restorations.

New technologies, such as airborne-particle abrasion devices, atraumatic restorative treatment (ART), chemo-mechanical caries removal, lasers, detector dyes, and negative air ion (NAI) systems, can increase the comfort and success of dental restorations, as well as increase the speed of their placement. However, marginal adaptation has continued to be an ongoing technical problem.

Reversal of PRCLs is associated with remineralization and a corresponding reduction in acidogenic and aciduric microorganisms.[12–16] Therefore, an antimicrobial method to manage PRCLs would be useful.[17] When lesions become inactive, ie, hard or arrested, they acquire a smooth and hard surface. It should be noted that in one study arrested lesions remained unchanged during several years of observation.[18]

The best management strategy for root caries still needs to be developed. The possibility of preventing and controlling root caries for all populations worldwide is a strong incentive. However, compared to enamel caries, there has been relatively limited research into the pharmaceutical management of root caries, and many of these studies have been carried out in vitro. As an alternative management strategy for root caries, ozone can be considered. Ozone has strong oxidation power and has been used for deodorization, decolorization, and oxidation. This powerful oxidant is also effective for the inactivation of microorganisms. The mechanism of microbial inactivation by ozone is thought to occur by general inactivation of the entire cell in microorganisms.

The Use of Ozone in Medicine

Ozone has been used in several medical applications.[19–30] Many studies have investigated the use of this therapy in the treatment of ocular diseases such as optic neuropathies, glaucoma, central retinal vein obstructions, and degenerative retinal diseases. Furthermore, in patients with myocardial infarction, endovenous ozone therapy has a beneficial effect on blood lipid metabolism, decreasing blood cholesterol and provoking the activation of antioxidant protection system.[31]

Ozone itself is not an oxygen radical, but it generates oxidants (reactive oxygen species [ROS]). This oxidant reacts with many blood components such as lipoproteins, plasma proteins, lymphocytes, monocytes, granulocytes, platelets, and erythrocytes. In a defense reaction to the generation of ROS, the various antioxidant systems are activated and go on to produce antioxidant enzymes and scavengers.[32] Since the oxidizing effect of ozone is almost linearly related to its concentration in the blood, above a certain threshold it becomes very cytotoxic and produces hemolysis. The half-life of ozone is short, and this oxidant rapidly converts into oxygen via an endothermic reaction. Ozone treatment can positively affect microcirculation. Some of the beneficial biologic effects of ozone in medical practice are the improvement of oxygen metabolism, the increase of cell energy, the immunomodulator property, and the enhancement of the antioxidant defense system.[20,33–35] The use of ozone therapy on age-related degenerative retinal maculopathy[35] demonstrated a decrease in lipid peroxidation but an increase in superoxide dismutase and an enzyme scavenger of anion superoxide. In this respect, ozone was able to minimize the damage produced by lipid peroxidation by increasing the antioxidant defense system.[36–39]

Studies on filterability of blood after ozone treatment showed an increase in membrane fluidity (MF) simultaneous with a reduction in sedimentation rate. In addition, ozonized blood was shown to have a protective effect on ischemia-reperfusion injury in different organs such as the liver, kidney, and brain. Shiratori et al[20] demonstrated that ozone treatment had a positive effect on energy charge (EC), and adenosine triphosphate (ATP) was well maintained in brain hypoxia. The authors also stated that lactate production was inhibited and survival time was significantly increased.

Interestingly, Zee and Monte reported on two nonsurgical patients who were suffering from chronic leg ulceration for 2 years and with whom conventional therapies failed (personal communication, 2001). Autohematherapy with ozone was the last option for these patients, whose legs were planned for amputation. Ozone was initially administered twice a week and had an immediate effect on swelling, edema, and the intensity of the pain. Healing was slow but steady. A complete healing of the ulcers was achieved following ozone treatment.

Ozone exerts its protective effects by means of an oxidative preconditioning, stimulation, and/or preservation of the endogenous antioxidant systems. Al-Dalain et al[40] reported the effects of ozone on the oxidative stress related to diabetes mellitus. In this study, ozone treatment improved glycemic control and prevented oxidative stress related to diabetes mellitus and its complications. Ozone protective effects on antioxidant endogenous defense also improved glucose metabolism in diabetic patients.

In another study, Copello et al[41] investigated the effect of ozone application in patients (n = 68) with retinitis pigmentosa, which is characterized by progressive night blindness, in a controlled, randomized, double-blind clinical trial. Patients were treated with ozone by rectal administration (dose = 10 mg) for 15 sessions. Copello et al[41] reported a significant improvement in 88.2% of patients treated with ozone compared with 23.5% in the control group and stated that it could be useful to apply ozone therapy in the first stage of retinitis pigmentosa and at 6-month intervals to enhance visual capabilities in patients with this disease.

Recently, Zamora et al[42] also reported the use of ozone for the management of septic shock (inflammatory response). In their study, groups pretreated with ozone and antibiotics in combination showed a significant increase of survival of rats in comparison with the groups treated only with antibiotics. The survival rate for the groups treated only with antibiotics were less than 25%. These results clearly showed that ozone was useful in the inflammatory response. Ozone pretreatment in combination with antibiotics was capable of reducing the mortality of the rats. The microorganisms have developed resistance to antibiotics, and so in the pharmaceutical field new germicidal products such as cephalosporine and quinolones are continuously being developed. Ozone applied prophylactically was able to increase or support the antibiotic action. Zamora et al[42] suggested that the prophylactic application of ozone may downregulate the inflammatory response and inhibit the expression of interleukin-1 in the liver.

The Use of Ozone in Dentistry

The preventive and therapeutic effects of ozone in medicine have been well established.[43] Unfortunately, very few studies have reported on the use of ozone for dental purposes.

Recently, there is growing concern regarding the quality of water that exits in dental unit waterlines. The numbers of microorganisms that have been found in water samples collected from dental units may exceed current limits for water quality and are perceived as a potential health risk to patients and dental personnel.[44–46] Fortunately, ozone has been successfully employed for the treatment of dental unit waterlines since the 1990s. The microbial effect of ozone on dental treatment units lasted longer than did that of conventional methods such as hydrogen peroxide/silver ion solutions in vivo and in vitro.[47–49] Filippi[50–55] tested the effect of ozone on *Pseudomonas aeruginosa*, a potentially pathogenic microorganism frequently found in dental treatment units. After treatment with 10 µg ozone/mL water, no microorganisms were detected in the water. Furthermore, there was no evidence of air pollution related to the use of ozone in the treatment area and no ozone detected in the water drawn from the dental waterlines.

Subsequently, ozonated water was considered to be an alternative to a sterile isotonic solution for oral rinse during dental surgery or following tooth extraction. Filippi found that ozonized water applied on a daily basis can accelerate the healing rate in oral mucosa. The effect was observed on the first two postoperative days. Between days 2 and 7 after surgery, there were no further effects observed related to ozone. However, the author observed that, under the influence of ozone, within the first 48 hours the final wound closure was modified, more wounds were closed after 7 days, and cell proliferation commenced earlier. The author stated that the use of ozone is completely safe because ozone dissipates very quickly in water. It was concluded that the influence of ozone led to a higher expression of cytokines, especially transforming growth factor (TGF)–α1, that were important for wound healing, as well as for regulation and coordination in the initial wound healing phase. TGF-α1 had a marked influence on cell proliferation, chemotaxis (monocytes and fibroblasts), angiogenesis, synthesis of extracellular matrix, and collagen synthesis. However, medically relevant properties of ozonated water in oral surgery still remain to be proved.

A denture cleaner using ozone bubbles (ozone concentration approximately 10 ppm) was considered to be clinically appropriate in view of its strong disinfecting and deodorizing power and its high biologic safety.[56] The effectiveness of this cleaner against *Candida albicans* was investigated, and levels of this microbe were found to decrease to about $^1/_{10}$ of their initial value after 30 minutes and to $^1/_{103}$ after 60 minutes of exposure. Subsequently, Suzuki et al[57] also examined the influence of ozone on the surface of removable partial denture alloys to determine its usefulness as a cleaning method for removable partial dentures. The researchers reported that ozone treatment caused a slight change in the gold-copper-silver-palladium alloy in terms of reflectance. However, the changes were significantly less than those caused by acid-electrolyzed water and a commercial denture cleaner.

However, no study has clinically evaluated the therapeutic benefits of ozone for the management of root caries. Recently Baysan et al[58] for the first time reported that ozone application either for 10 or 20 seconds effectively killed the great majority of microorganisms in PRCLs in vitro by the employment of a novel ozone delivery

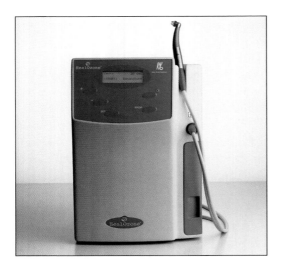

Fig 7-1 HealOzone delivery system. (Courtesy of KaVo, Biberach, Germany.)

system (HealOzone). A 10-second application was also capable of reducing the numbers of *Streptococcus mutans* and *S sobrinus* in vitro.

The authors of this chapter believe that the use of ozone in dentistry is conservative and harmless. This proposed ozone delivery system is being investigated in in vitro and in vivo studies. Recent clinical studies have reported on the effect of ozone on the microbial flora and clinical severity of primary root caries by the ozone delivery system.[59–62] In addition, the same authors have investigated the safety and efficacy of ozone use for the management of root caries in a longitudinal study. Two clinical studies from this investigation are reported below.

Clinical Study 1

In this study, the ozone delivery system (HealOzone) that was employed is a portable apparatus for the treatment of caries. It can deliver ozone at a concentration of 2,100 ppm ± 10%. The vacuum pump pulls air at 615 cc/min through the generator to supply ozone to the lesion and purges the system of ozone after the treatment. A disposable removable silicone cup, attached to the handpiece, is provided for receiving the gas and exposing a selected area of the tooth to the gas. The tightly fitting cup seals the selected area on the tooth to prevent escape of ozone (Fig 7-1).

The data for this study have been obtained from a total of 70 PRCLs in 26 patients. Each PRCL was classified subjectively in terms of color, texture, cavitation, size, hardness, and severity. Leathery lesions with a severity index of 1 or 2 were selected; they corresponded to the perceived treatment need index categories deemed to require a pharmaceutical approach or caries removal only, respectively.[12] PRCLs were exposed to the ozone gas for either 10 or 20 seconds. After the ozone application, each subject was recalled between 3 and 5.5 months for investigation of any adverse events with a

Table 7-1 Mean ± SE $\log_{10}$ (cfu + 1) and $\log_{10}$ (cfu + 1)/mg before and after 10- and 20-second ozone application*

Groups	$\log_{10}$ (cfu + 1)		$\log_{10}$ (cfu + 1)/mg	
	10 s	20 s	10 s	20 s
Control samples	7.00 ± 0.24	6.00 ± 0.21	7.92 ± 0.23	7.04 ± 0.23
Ozonated samples	4.35 ± 0.49	0.46 ± 0.26	5.04 ± 0.56	1.26 ± 0.48

*$P < .001$

detailed questionnaire and reassessment of the severity of the PRCLs.

Reduction in Total Microorganisms

The total cultivable microflora was assessed by counts of the colony-forming units (cfu) recovered. The colony-forming units were divided by the samples' weights. There was a significant ($P < .001$) difference between the control and test samples for either 10 or 20 seconds in $\log_{10}$ (cfu + 1) shown per milligram (Table 7-1).

Statistical Analyses

Microbiological counts from test and control groups for each study were transformed as $\log_{10}$ (cfu + 1) prior to statistical analyses in order to normalize their distributions and ensure group variance homogeneity. Statistical analyses of the data were obtained by paired Student t tests to determine differences between test and control groups; the threshold of significance chosen was 0.05. Means and standard errors were also recorded. Pearson's correlation coefficients were performed to evaluate the significance of correlations between the reduction in total microorganisms and the clinical detection criteria used to detect PRCLs. Analysis of variance (ANOVA) followed by Duncan's multiple range tests were also used to assess differences between the reduction of total microorganisms after treating test samples with ozone for a period of either 10 or 20 seconds and severity indices 1 and 2. All analyses were performed using the SPSS statistical package for Microsoft Windows version 6.1.

Color

Color of PRCLs failed to correlate with the reduction of microorganisms after ozone application for either 10 or 20 seconds.

Cavitation

Cavitation was estimated as the greatest loss of tooth structure between the lesion surface and the original contour of the tooth. Using Pearson's correlation test, there was a significant ($P < .05$) correlation between cavitation and reduction in total microorganisms after ozone application for 10 seconds ($r = 0.39$) (Fig 7-2). Reduction in total microorganisms after ozone application for 20 seconds failed to correlate with cavitation ($r = 0.22$).

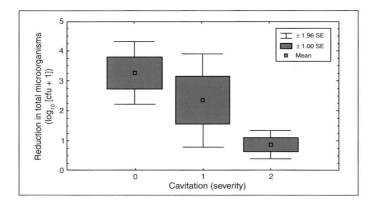

Fig 7-2 Correlation of reduction in total microorganisms with cavitation of PRCLs after ozone application for 10 seconds ($P < .05$). Severity of cavitation was rated according to the perceived treatment need index.

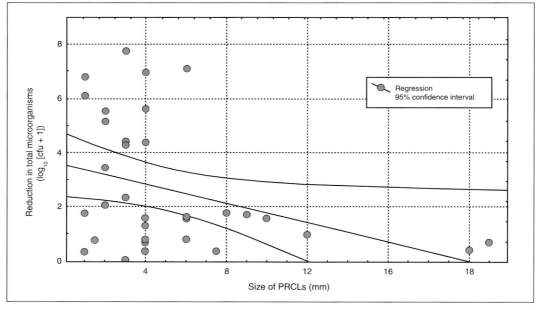

Fig 7-3 Correlation of reduction in total microorganisms with the size of PRCLs after ozone application for 10 seconds ($r = 0.44$).

Size

The size of each lesion was estimated by multiplying the height of the lesion by its width. Using Pearson's correlation test, reduction in total microorganisms after ozone application for 10 seconds corre-

lated with the size of PRCLs ($r = 0.44$) (Fig 7-3). Smaller lesions presented a greater reduction in total microorganisms following ozone application than did larger lesions. Reduction in total microorganisms after ozone application for 20 seconds failed to correlate with size ($r = 0.05$).

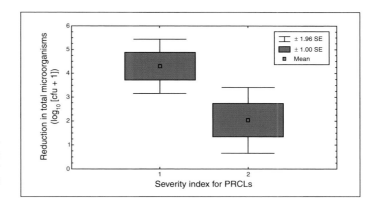

Fig 7-4 Reduction in total microorganisms related to the severity indices of PRCLs after ozone application for 10 seconds ($P < .05$).

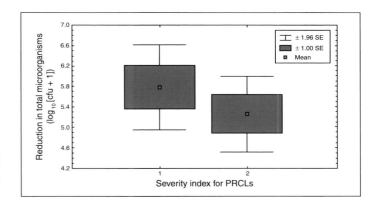

Fig 7-5 Reduction in total microorganisms related to the severity indices of PRCLs after ozone application for 20 seconds ($P < .05$).

Hardness

All lesions were of a leathery consistency before ozone treatment. After application of ozone for 10 seconds, 7 (22%) of the 33 lesions had become hard compared with 26 (81%) of the 32 lesions after 20 seconds of ozone application.

Distance from the Gingival Margin

Using Pearson's correlation test, reduction in total microorganisms after ozone application for 10 seconds correlated with the distance of PRCLs from the gingival margin ($r = 0.36$). Following ozone application, lesions that were far from the gingival margin exhibited greater reduction in total microorganisms than did the lesions closer to the gingival margin. Reduction in total microorganisms after ozone application for 20 seconds failed to correlate with the distance of PRCLs from the gingival margin ($r = 0.24$).

Severity Index

Using ANOVA followed by Duncan's multiple range tests, reduction of total microorganisms after ozone application on test samples for either 10 or 20 seconds showed significant differences between severity indices 1 and 2 ($P < .05$) (Figs 7-4 and 7-5). The reduction in total microorganisms in clinical severity index 1 was significantly greater than was the reduction in total microorganisms in clinical severity index 2. Pearson's correlation test also showed a clear relationship between the reduction of total microorganisms and clinical severity indices 1 and 2 for PRCLs ($r = 0.48$).

Clinical Study 2

In this study, all participants were patients attending Queen's University School of Dentistry in Belfast, Northern Ireland, for routine oral health care. Each subject had given informed consent for both dental examinations and ozone treatment. The data for this study has been obtained from a total of 100 PRCLs in 50 patients. The ozone delivery system described in clinical study 1 was employed.

The following are the inclusion criteria for subjects in this clinical study:

- Male or female at least 18 years of age.
- Root carious lesions deemed to require caries removal in the middle severity category (category 2; leathery: debride) on at least two surfaces and that are accessible for the diagnostic procedure.
- Written informed consent for this protocol obtained prior to study enrollment. Each subject was required to sign and date the informed consent form prior to participation.

The following are the exclusion criteria for subjects in this clinical study:

- Fewer than two active root carious lesions in the middle severity category (category 2; leathery: debride).

- Presence of advanced periodontal disease in the test tooth with a PRCL (eg, purulent exudate, tooth mobility, and/or extensive bone loss).
- Participation in another dental study during the previous 3 months.
- Any condition that, in the opinion of the investigator, would preclude participation by the subject (such as cross-infection control risk).

Reassessment of the Severity of PRCLs

Out of the 65 PRCLs reviewed, 33 lesions had become hard, 27 lesions reversed to severity index 1 from severity index 2, and 5 lesions remained the same following ozone application for either 10 or 20 seconds. The breakdown of root caries severity classification at baseline and recall are shown in Table 7-2. Two objective methods were used to measure severity: an electrical caries monitor and a laser-based caries detection device.

Electrical caries monitor

The electrical caries monitor ECM III (Lode Diagnostics, Groningen, The Netherlands) was used to measure the electrical resistance of each carious lesion. The ECM measures the electrical resistance of a site on the tooth during controlled drying. When the surface is dry, the resistance is determined by the tooth structure, and short circuiting to the soft tissues by the surface liquid (saliva) is avoided. The electrical resistance was measured at 23.3 Hz and less than 0.3 µA while the tooth was kept dry for 5 seconds with an air flow rate of 5.1 min.$^{-1}$ During the ECM readings, the measuring probe was applied to a lesion while the

Table 7-2 Cross tabulation of root caries severity classification on recalls after ozone application for either 10 or 20 seconds

Time	Before ozone application	After ozone application		
		Hard	SI 1	SI 2
10 s	SI 1 (n = 11)	6 (55%)	5 (45%)	0
	SI 2 (n = 22)	1 (5%)	21 (95%)	0
20 s	SI 1 (n = 7)	7 (100%)	0	0
	SI 2 (n = 25)	19 (76%)	6 (24%)	0

SI=Severity index

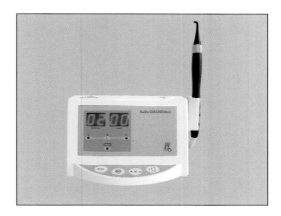

Fig 7-6 DIAGNOdent system (Courtesy of KaVo, Biberach, Germany).

subject held the reference electrode. Measurements were taken at the center, mesial, distal, occlusal, and gingival points of each root carious lesion. The monitor recorded the value at the end of the drying period (end value) and the area under the curve during the drying period (integrated value).

DIAGNOdent system

A laser-based device (DIAGNOdent, KaVo) was recently introduced and tested for its effectiveness in detecting occlusal caries in vitro (Fig 7-6).[63] The diagnostic accuracy of DIAGNOdent to detect occlusal caries was significantly better than that of radiography (P < .001) under in vitro conditions.[64] Validation studies and studies on repeatability and reproducibility should be performed in vivo before large-scale application of this device. Shi et al[65] reported a validation and comparison study on quantitative light-induced fluorescence (QLF) and DIAGNOdent for the quantification of smooth-surface caries and concluded that the correlation with the lesion depth was similar for the two methods tested (r = 0.85). However, the correlation with the mineral loss was higher for QLF than for DIAGNOdent ($r = 0.76$ and 0.67, respectively). It should be noted that there is limited data available to assess the efficacy of DIAGNOdent for the detection of root caries, especially early carious lesions.

In this study, step-by-step calibration was performed using tip "A" from the manufacturer for each session. Measurements were taken at the center, mesial, distal, occlusal, and gingival points of each root carious lesion. This recorded the numerical values. The mean of the five readings was used for statistical analyses.

Clinical assessments of both groups were undertaken at baseline and after 1 and 3 months. Medical and dental histories were recorded. The study involved patients with two PRCLs, and they were randomly allocated to one of the two groups. For the test group ozone was applied to the PRCLs for 10 seconds at baseline and after 3 months. The groups were as follows:

Group 1

The electrical resistance (via employment of the ECM) and DIAGNOdent measurements of each PRCL were determined. Subsequently, clinical criteria used to detect PRCLs were evaluated.[59] After cleaning with a sterile toothbrush and water, the tooth surface was isolated and dried with sterile cotton-wool rolls. Ozone was then delivered for 10 seconds into the cup, which was closely adapted to each PRCL. As part of the suction system, captured residual ozone was passed from the delivery system through manganese ions, which acted as an ozone destructor. The dental unit high-speed suction sys-

tem was also used on every occasion. PRCLs were not removed following ozone application. After 1 and 3 months, the electrical resistance and DIAGNOdent measurements and clinical criteria used to detect PRCLs were again examined. Ozone application was omitted.

Group 2

The electrical resistance and DIAGNOdent measurements and clinical criteria to detect PRCLs were evaluated. Ozone treatment was not performed on lesions in group 2 subjects. After 1 and 3 months, the electrical resistance and DIAGNOdent measurements and clinical criteria used to detect PRCLs were examined. Ozone application was again omitted.

Patients in both groups received full preventive instruction, including extensive oral hygiene and dietary advice, together with that concerning the use of the 1,100 ppm fluoride-containing dentifrice.

Readings from the ECM

At baseline, the ECM readings were similar for both groups. The mean ECM readings for the control group were similar to baseline readings after 1 and 3 months. In contrast, the mean ECM readings of the lesions in the ozone group increased after 1 and 3 months (Fig 7-7). There were statistically significant differences in the changes in ECM readings between the two groups after 1 and 3 months ($P < .001$). The greatest improvements in ECM measurements were in those lesions that were noncavitated at baseline, compared with lesions that were cavitated.

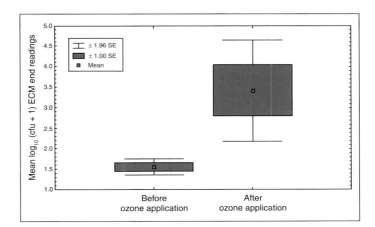

Fig 7-7 Mean $\log_{10}$ (cfu + 1) ECM end readings before and after ozone application for 10 seconds ($P < .001$).

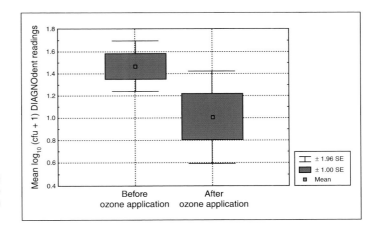

Fig 7-8 Mean $\log_{10}$ (cfu + 1) DIAGNOdent readings before and after ozone application for 10 seconds ($P < .01$).

Readings from the DIAGNOdent System

At baseline, the DIAGNOdent readings were similar for both groups. The mean DIAGNOdent readings for the control group were similar to baseline readings after 1 and 3 months. However, the mean DIAGNOdent readings of the lesions in the ozone group decreased after 1 and 3 months (Fig 7-8). There were statistically significant differences in the changes in DIAGNOdent readings between the two groups after 1 and 3 months ($P < .001$).

Ozone Application versus Conventional Treatments

The main clinical problem with the pharmaceutical approach for the management of root caries is the difficulty in suppressing or eliminating acidogenic and aciduric microorganisms for extended

109

periods. After treatment with a pharmaceutical approach, organisms may proliferate and recolonize in PRCLs. In the two studies described above, most of the PRCLs had become hard or had reversed to a less severe status after ozone application. It can be speculated that this reversal is associated with several factors, including the biopsy for the microbiologic samples, the microbial reduction, and the oxidant effects on PRCLs. The ecologic niche of the acidogenic and aciduric microorganisms will have been virtually eradicated from the microbial flora. This shifting of microbial flora to the normal oral commensals would mostly allow remineralization to occur within the carious process.

In addition, the oxidant sodium hypochlorite has previously been shown to improve the remineralization potential of demineralized dentin. Inaba et al[66] found that the use of an oxidant (10% sodium hypochlorite) on demineralized root dentin lesions improved their potential to remineralize, because sodium hypochlorite is a nonspecific proteolytic agent and can effectively remove organic components in the lesions. Subsequently, Inaba et al[67] showed that when the root dentin samples were treated with this oxidant for 2 minutes, permeability of fluoride ions increased. They concluded that removal of the organic materials from the dentin lesions was an acceptable approach to enhance remineralization. This may partly account for the dramatic remineralization seen after ozone application in these studies. However, ozone is a much more powerful oxidant than sodium hypochlorite.[59]

After the initial suppression of the numbers of total microorganisms, recolonization of the microorganisms may be retarded by a resistance of the commensal normal oral flora against intruding organisms into lesions.[68] In addition, the ecologic niche of these acidogenic and aciduric microorganisms would be severely disrupted, which in turn could interfere with recolonization by this specific microflora. Therefore, this may result in long-term suppression of acidogenic and aciduric microorganisms in PRCLs. Emilson et al[69] also reported that after a short-term intensive treatment of the dentition with chlorhexidine, *S mutans* was suppressed in vivo for a significant length of time (14 weeks).

Ozone has been employed in medicine since the 1950s. It has been estimated that more than 10 million people (primarily in Germany, Russia, and Cuba) have been given biooxidative therapies over the past 70 years to treat more than 50 different diseases. They include heart and blood vessel diseases, lung diseases, infectious diseases, and immune-related disorders. In addition, ozone had a very limited application in buildings for the elimination of microorganisms for many years. It is now accepted as a beneficial odor eliminator in restaurants, kitchens, homes, etc. The US Occupational Safety and Health Administration (OSHA) has established acceptable levels of ozone at 0.10 ppm for indoor air and 0.12 ppm for ambient air. Ozonation is recognized as an environmentally safe and effective process for the treatment of industrial effluents, drinking water, and sewage. In addition, Baysan and Lynch observed no adverse events during and after their clinical studies.[59]

Restorative materials fail at alarming rates, costing patients in terms of pain, discomfort, and finances. In England and Wales, a total of £1.5 billion were spent on

National Health Service (NHS) dentistry in general dental practice alone for dental treatment in 2000.[70] This does not include private treatment in England and Wales, which is currently estimated to be in excess of 50% of the clinicians' fees. In addition, hospitals and community dental clinics have enormous budgets for dental care of patients, certainly hundreds of millions of pounds annually. Therefore, the real cost of dental treatment in England and Wales exceeded £3 billion in 2000. Most of these fees are due to restorations, root obturations, dentures, crowns, and fixed partial dentures. A substantial portion of the costs for periodontal treatments are associated with iatrogenic aspects of treating caries. Clearly, the use of ozone instead of restorations to treat caries can save billions of pounds in the United Kingdom alone, not to mention the absence of pain, discomfort, and time off work that is associated with ozone treatment.

In addition to the obvious failures associated with dental restorations for the management of root caries, many problems arise directly related to the conventional method of "drilling and filling," eg, pain caused by the injection of anesthetic both during tooth preparation and afterward (some patients experience trismus and hematomas as a direct result of injection). During tooth preparation, a handpiece is used, often with a diamond bur rotating at hundreds of thousands of revolutions per minute, which can sometimes result in severe damage to the oral soft tissues. This can be associated with inadvertent movement of the patient and may damage nerves and soft tissues (every year clinicians are sued as a result of severing the lingual nerve, which can occur during tooth preparation). Pulpal damage may also occur as a result of the dessication and heating of the pulpal contents, possibly causing irreversible damage to the pulp that may then require either root canal therapy or tooth extraction. Common adverse effects also include tooth sensitivity because all resin composite restorative materials shrink on setting, leaving small gaps around the restoration that sometimes induce sensitivity to heat, cold, or even osmotic changes. Furthermore, medically compromised patients (eg, patients with infective endocarditis or bleeding disorders, those taking steroids) can be at risk of death as a result of conventional local anesthesia, tooth preparation, and restoration. Ozone treatment does not involve these risks.

In conclusion, the economic consequences of simpler and less prolonged dental treatment would also be beneficial because treatment times are reduced. In the past, cost analysis was based principally on the comparative market price of new treatment compared with standard therapy. Benefits were assessed solely in terms of objective clinical improvement. Now, issues such as quality of life, early return to occupation, and subjective symptoms of pain and discomfort caused by a treatment are also being critically evaluated.[71–73] Ozone application can be performed effectively and safely for the management of root caries as an alternative to conventional restorative treatments.

Acknowledgment

The authors wish to thank Dr Robert Whiley for his support with the microbiologic analyses.

References

1. Pine CM, Pitts NB, Steele JG, Nunn JN, Treasure E. Dental restorations in adults in the UK in 1998 and implications for the future. Br Dent J 2001;190:4–8.

2. Lynch E, Tay WM. Glass-ionomer cements. Part 3. Clinical properties II. J Irish Dent Assoc 1989; 35:66–73.

3. Seichter U. Root surface caries: A critical literature review. J Am Dent Assoc 1987;115:305–310.

4. Takahashi K, Emilson CG, Birkhed D. Fluoride release in vitro from various glass-ionomer cements and resin composites after exposure to NaF solutions. Dent Mater 1993;9:350–354.

5. Dijkman GE, de Vries J, Arends J. Secondary caries in dentine around composites: A wavelength-independent microradiographical study. Caries Res 1994;28:87–93.

6. Vermeersch G, Leloup G, Vreven J. Fluoride release from glass-ionomer cements, compomers and resin composites. J Oral Rehabil 2001;28: 26–32.

7. Torli Y, Itota T, Okamoto M, Nakabo S, Nagamine M, Inoue K. Inhibition of artificial secondary caries in roots by fluoride-releasing restorative materials. Oper Dent 2001;26:36–43.

8. Qvist V, Qvist J, Mjör IA. Placement and longevity of tooth-colored restorations in Denmark. Acta Odontol Scand 1990;48:305–311.

9. Elderton RJ. Treating restorative dentistry to health. Br Dent J 1996;181:221–225.

10. Bowen RL, Marjennhoff WA. Dental composites/glass ionomers: The materials. Adv Dent Res 1992;6:44–49.

11. Yip KH, Peng D, Smales RJ. Effects of APF gel on the physical structure of compomers and glass-ionomer cements. Oper Dent 2001;26:231–238.

12. Beighton D, Lynch E, Heath MR. A microbiological study of primary root caries lesions with different treatment needs. J Dent Res 1993; 73:623–629.

13. Lynch E, Beighton D. Relationships between mutans streptococci and perceived treatment need of primary root-caries lesions. Gerodontology 1993;10:98–104.

14. Schüppach P, Osterwalder V, Gunnenheim B. Human root caries: Microbiota in plaque covering sound, carious and arrested carious root surfaces. Caries Res 1995;29:382–395.

15. Lynch E. Relationships Between Clinical Criteria and Microflora of Primary Root Caries. [Proceedings of the First Annual Indiana Conference, Indianapolis, 1995]. Indianapolis, IN: Indiana University School of Dentistry, 1996:195–242.

16. Lynch E. The Diagnosis and Management of Primary Root Caries [thesis]. London: University of London, 1994.

17. Lynch E. Antimicrobial management of primary root carious lesions. Gerodontol 1996;13: 118–129.

18. Papas AS, Palmer CA, McGandy RB, Hartz SC, Russell RM. Dietary and nutritional factors in relation to dental caries in elderly subjects. Gerodontics 1987;3:30–37.

19. Belianin II, Shmelev E. The use of an ozonized sorbent in treating patients with progressive pulmonary tuberculosis combined with hepatitis [in Russian]. Ter Arkh 1994;66:29–32.

20. Shiratori R, Kaneko Y, Kobayashi Y, et al. Can ozone administration activate the tissue metabolism? A study on brain metabolism during hypoxic hypoxia [in Japanese]. Masui 1993;42:2–6.

21. Paulesu L, Luzi E, Bocci V. Studies on the biological effects of ozone: 2. Induction of tumor necrosis factor (TNF-alpha) on human leukocytes. Lymphokine Cytokine Res 1991;10:409–412.

22. Bocci V. Autohaemotherapy after treatment of blood with ozone. A reappraisal. J Int Med Res 1994;22:131–144.

23. Riva Sanseverino E, Castellacci P, Misciali C, Borrello P, Venturo N. Effects of ozonised autohaemotherapy on human hair cycle [in Italian]. Panminerva Medica 1995;37:129–132.

24. Cooke ED, Pockley AG, Tucker AT, Kirby JD, Bolton AE. Treatment of severe Raynaud's syndrome by injection of autologous blood pretreated by heating, ozonation and exposure to ultraviolet light (H-O-U) therapy. Int Angiol 1997;16:250–254.

25. Ozmen V, Thomas WO, Healy JT, et al. Irrigation of the abdominal cavity in the treatment of experimentally induced microbial peritonitis: Efficacy of ozonated saline. Am Surg 1993;59: 297–303.

26. Romero Valdes A, Blanco Gonzales R, Menendez Cepero S, Gomez Moraleda M, Ley Pozo J. Arteriosclerosis obliterans and ozone therapy. Its administration by different routes [in Spanish]. Angiologia 1993;45:177–179.

27. Rodriquez MM, Garcia J, Menendez S, Devesa E, Gonzalez R. Ozone medical application in the treatment of senile dementia. Ozone in Medicine. Presented at the 2nd International Symposium on Ozone Application, Havana, Cuba, 1997.

28. Dolphin S, Walker M. Healing accelerated by ionozone therapy. Physiotherapy 1979;65:81–82.

29. Gloor M, Lipphardt BA. Studies on ozone therapy of acne vulgaris [in German]. Z Hautkr 1976; 51:97–101.

30. D'erme M, Scarchilli A, Artale AM, Pasquali Lasagni M. Ozone therapy in lumbar sciatic pain [in Italian]. Radiol Med (Torino) 1998;95:21–24.

31. Hernandez F, Menendez S, Wong R. Decrease of blood cholesterol and stimulation of antioxidative response in cardiopathy patients treated with endovenous ozone therapy. Free Radic Biol Med 1995;19:115–119.

32. Bocci V. Biological and clinical effects of ozone. Has ozone therapy a future in medicine? Br J Biomed Sci 1999;56:270–279.

33. Viebahn-Haensler R. The Use of Ozone in Medicine, ed 3. Iffezheim, Germany: ODREI-Publishers, 1999:95–119.

34. Bocci V. Ozone as a bioregulator. Pharmacology and toxicology of ozonetherapy today. J Biol Regul Homeost Agents 1996;10:31–53.

35. Barber E, Menendez S, Ledn OS, et al. Prevention of renal injury after induction of ozone tolerance in rats submitted to warm ischaemia. Mediators Inflamm 1999;8:37–41.

36. León OS, Menendez S, Merino N, et al. Ozone oxidative preconditioning: A protection against cellular damage by free radicals. Mediators Inflamm 1998;7:289–294.

37. Peralta C, León OS, Xaus C, et al. Protective effect of ozone treatment on the injury associated with hepatic ischemia-reperfusion: Antioxidant-prooxidant balance. Free Radic Res 1999;31: 191–196.

38. Candelario-Jalil E, Mohammed-Al-Dalain S, Fernandez OS, et al. Oxidative preconditioning affords protection against carbon tetrachloride–induced glycogen depletion and oxidative stress in rats. J Appl Toxicol 2001;21:297–301.

39. Riva Sanseverino E, Meduri RA, Pizzino A, Prantera M, Martini E. Effects of oxygen-ozone therapy on age-related degenerative retinal maculopathy [in Italian]. Panminerva Med 1990;32:77–84.

40. Al-Dalain SM, Martinez G, Candelario-Jalil E, et al. Ozone treatment reduces markers of oxidative and endothelial damage in an experimental diabetes model in rats. Pharmacol Res 2001; 44:391–396.

41. Copello M, Eguia F, Menendez S, Menendez H. Ozone therapy in patients with retinitis pigmentosa. Presented at the 15th Annual Ozone World Congress, London, 14 Sept 2001.

42. Zamora ZB, Menendez S, Bette M, Mutters R, Hoffmann S, Schulz S. Ozone Prophylactic Effect and Antibiotics as a Modulator of Inflammatory Septic Process in Rats. In: Proceedings of the 15th Annual Ozone World Congress. London: International Ozone Association, 2001:202–211.

43. Baysan A, Lynch E, Grootveld M. The use of ozone for the management of primary root carious lesions. In: Albrektsson TO, Bratthall D, Glantz POJ, Lindhe JT (eds). Tissue Preservation in Caries Treatment. Chicago: Quintessence, 2001:49–67.

44. Barbeau J, Tanguay R, Faucher E, et al. Multiparametric analysis of water line contamination of dental units. Appl Environ Microbiol 1996;62: 3954–3959.

45. Williams JF, Johnston AM, Johnson B, Huntington MK, Mackenzie CD. Microbial contamination of dental unit waterlines: Prevalence, intensity and microbiological characteristics. J Am Dent Assoc 1993;124:59–65.

46. Putnins EE, Di Giovanni D, Bhullar AS. Dental unit waterline contamination and its possible implications during periodontal surgery. J Periodontol 2001;72:393–400.

47. Lee TK, Waked EJ, Wolinsky LE, Mito RS, Danielson RE. Controlling biofilm and microbial contamination in dental unit waterlines. J Calif Dent Assoc 2001;29:679–684.

48. Filippi A, Tilkes F, Beck KG, Kirschner H. Water disinfection of dental treatment units using ozone. Dtsch Zahnarztl Z 1991;46:485–487.

49. Filippi A. Bewährung der Wasserdesinfektion zahnärztlicher Behandlungseinheiten durch Ozon. Dtsch Zahnärztl Z 1995;50:708–710.

50. Filippi A. Ozone is the most effective disinfectant for dental treatment units: Results after 8 years of comparison. Ozone Sci Eng 1997;19: 527–532

51. Filippi A. Ozone in oral surgery—Current status and prospects. Ozone Sci Eng 1997;19:387–393.

52. Filippi A. Ozone in the room air when using water ozonating equipment in the dental treatment area. Ozone Sci Eng 1998;20:251–257.

53. Filippi A. Ozoniertes Wasser als Kühl- und Spülmedium bei Osteotomie. Dtsch Zahnärztl Z 1999;54:619–622.

54. Filippi A. The influence of the water heater in dental chairs on the ozone concentration in the water used. Ozone Sci Eng 1999;21:629–633.

55. Filippi A. The influence of ozonised water on the epithelial wound healing process in the oral cavity. In: Proceedings of the 15th Ozone World Congress. London: International Ozone Association, 2001:212–220.

56. Murakami H, Sakuma S, Nakamura K, et al. Disinfection of removable dentures using ozone. Dent Mater J 1996;15:220–225.

57. Suzuki T, Oizumi M, Furuya J, Okamoto Y, Rosenstiel SF. Influence of ozone on oxidation of dental alloys. Int J Prosthodont 1999;12:179–183.

58. Baysan A, Whiley RA, Lynch E. Anti-microbial effect of a novel ozone-generating device on micro-organisms associated with primary root carious lesions in vitro. Caries Res 2000;34:498–501.

59. Baysan A, Lynch E. Effect of ozone on the microbial flora and clinical severity of primary root caries. Amer J Dent 2004;17:56–60.

60. Holmes J. Clinical reversal of root caries using ozone, double blind, randomized, controlled 18-month trial. Gerodontology 2003;20:106–114.

61. Baysan A, Prinz JF, Lynch E. Clinical criteria used to detect primary root caries with electrical and mechanical measurements in vitro. Am J Dent 2004;17:94–98.

62. Baysan A. Management of root caries using fluoride or ozone [thesis]. London: Univ of London, 2002.

63. Lussi A, Imwinkelried S, Pitts N, Longbottom C, Reich E. Performance and reproducibility of a laser fluorescence system for detection of occlusal caries in vitro. Caries Res 1999;33:261–266.

64. Shi XQ, Tranaeus S, Angmar-Mansson B. Validation of DIAGNOdent for quantification of smooth-surface caries: An in vitro study. Acta Odontol Scand 2001;59:74–78.

65. Shi XQ, Tranaeus S, Angmar-Mansson B. Comparison of QLF and DIAGNOdent for quantification of smooth-surface caries. Caries Res 2001;35:21–26.

66. Inaba D, Duschner H, Jongebloed W, Odelius H, Takagi O, Arends J. The effects of a sodium hypochlorite treatment on demineralized root dentin. Eur J Oral Sci 1995;103:368–374.

67. Inaba D, Ruben J, Takagi O, Arends J. Effects of sodium hypochlorite treatment on remineralization of human root dentine in vitro. Caries Res 1996;30:214–218.

68. Emilson CG. Effects of chlorhexidine gel treatment on Streptococcus mutans population in human saliva and dental plaque. Scand J Dent Res 1981;89:239–246.

69. Emilson CG, Ravald N, Birkhed D. Effects of a 12-month prophylactic programme on selected oral bacterial populations on root surfaces with active and inactive carious lesions. Caries Res 1993;27:195–200.

70. Dental Data Services. General Dental Council Annual Statistics: Gross Fees; April 1999–March 2000 in England and Wales. East Sussex, UK: Dental Practice Board, 2000.

71. Bowling A, Stramer K, Dickinson E, Windsor J, Bond M. Evaluation of specialists' outreach clinics in general practice in England: Process and acceptability to patients, specialists and general practitioners. J Epidemiol Community Health 1997;51:52–61.

72. Rubin H, Gandek B, Rogers W, Kosinski M, McHorney C, Ware J. Patients ratings of outpatients visits in different practice settings: Results from the medical outcomes study. J Am Med Assoc 1993;270:835–840.

73. Osborne D, Croucher R. Levels of burnout in general dental practitioners in the south-east of England. Br Dent J 1994;177:372–377.

Chapter 8

Are Adhesive Technologies Needed to Support Ceramics? An Assessment of the Current Evidence

F. J. Trevor Burke, Garry J. P. Fleming,
Dan Nathanson, Peter M. Marquis

Abstract

All-ceramic crowns offer the potential for increased esthetics compared with metal-ceramic crowns. Dental ceramics employed for all-ceramic restorations also resist wear extremely well and do not elicit a pulpal response from vital teeth as is common with some non-precious alloys used for metal-ceramic crown reconstruction. It can be seen from both laboratory testing data on the influence of cement type on specimen longevity and clinical studies on the failure rates of conventionally and adhesively luted crowns that when the placement procedure incorporates a dentin bonding step, enhanced survival rates are recorded. The laboratory fracture studies comparing restorations luted conventionally and adhesively, combined with the clinical and laboratory studies examining the strengthening of ceramics by the application of an adhesive lute compared with a conventional acid-base lute, would possibly preclude the use of nonadhesive technologies to support dental ceramics.

In dental clinical practice, crowns may be placed for a variety of reasons, principally the loss of tooth substance as a result of caries or trauma. For anterior teeth, good esthetics is essential, but resistance to fracture is also an important prerequisite. Porcelain, either alone or supported by metal, has been one of the materials used over the past four decades, with metal-ceramic crowns having been employed successfully in dentistry since they were first patented by Weinstein and coworkers[1] in 1962.

However, metal-ceramic crowns may exhibit less-than-ideal esthetics, because the gray metal core must be camouflaged with an opaque layer of ceramic. Only with difficulty can the limited translucency of metal-ceramic crowns replicate that of natural tooth substance.

Additionally, crowns may be in close proximity to the gingivae or may extend subgingivally. Elements from the alloy may be released in close proximity to the gingival tissue and may reach high concentrations in that area because they are not diluted by saliva.[2] The combination of suboptimal esthetics and the potential for sensitization of the gingival tissues has led the dental profession to examine methods for perfecting the all-ceramic crown as a possible replacement for metal-ceramic crowns.

In 1903,[3,4] Land developed a method for constructing an all-porcelain jacket crown. The same method is used today, although improvements have been made in the materials and techniques employed.[5] The low-strength ceramics employed by Land were of limited clinical use due to their susceptibility to fracture under masticatory load. To strengthen dental porcelain, it must either be supported by a high-strength substructure or the porcelain itself must be made stronger.[6] Alternatively, the ceramic may be supported by metal or the tooth itself. The application of veneering porcelains to high-strength ceramics was considered impractical because high-strength ceramics are opaque and not tooth-colored, unless extremely fine, submicron grains are used, the achievement of which is technically very demanding.[7] Additionally, mismatched thermal expansion coefficients may result in delamination of the veneering porcelain on firing. However, as dental ceramics tend to fail at a critical strain rate of 0.1%,[8] increased strength in ceramics can only be achieved by increasing the elastic modulus. Consequently, much of the research in the mid-1960s

was directed toward producing stronger restorations.

Methods of Improving the Strength of Ceramic Materials

A variety of methods have been used over the past four decades to attempt to improve the strength of ceramic materials.

Dispersion Strengthening

Binns[9] heat-pressed mixtures of alumina or zirconia crystals with different glasses. His results indicated that an increase in strength was obtained with an increased proportion of dispersed ceramic crystal—in the absence of a sudden volume change associated with the crystal structure or a difference in the thermal expansion coefficients between the glass and the dispersed ceramic inclusion. The author identified that, for a crack to propagate in a composite system where the thermal expansion coefficients of both the glassy matrix and inclusion crystals were similar and a good interface had formed, the fracture path traveled indiscriminately through both glass and crystal phases. In such a system, the higher strength and elasticity of the inclusion crystals carry a greater proportion of the load, and the energy required to fracture the composite material was greater than that for the glass alone (Fig 8-1).

Austin et al[11] found that by replacing up to 40% of the potter's flint in traditional whiteware bodies with a corresponding amount of 10-μm calcined alumina, the transverse strength of the whiteware was increased by up to 200%. Based on this finding and the results of

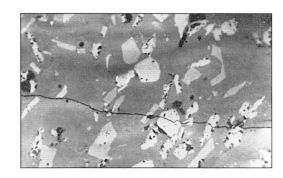

Fig 8-1 A two-phase crystal glass system in which the inclusion of 40% to 50% alumina crystals were employed as the reinforcing phase. The thermal expansion coefficients of both the glassy matrix and the inclusion crystals were similar so that the fracture path traveled indiscriminately through both the glass and the inclusion crystals. (Adapted from McLean and Hughes.[10])

the investigation by McLean and Hughes[10] of candidate ceramic oxide materials for dispersion strengthening of dental porcelain, McLean[12] selected alumina as having the greatest number of advantages. He stated that "there seemed little doubt that the mechanical properties of dental porcelain could be much improved by the inclusion of alumina crystals of high strength and elasticity." The results of mechanical tests by McLean and Hughes[10] showed that for a two-phase crystal glass system, in which the inclusion of 40% to 50% alumina crystals were employed as the reinforcing phase, the transverse bending strength was doubled compared with conventional feldspathic porcelain. The authors also found that for the two-phase crystal glass system the firing shrinkage was reduced and the resistance to thermal shock on cooling from firing temperature was increased when compared with conventional feldspathic porcelain. The practical use of aluminous core porcelain as the main reinforcement for porcelain jacket crowns was described by McLean,[12] and it is this system that is still frequently used today in the construction of all-porcelain jacket crowns.

McLean[6] reported a 2.1% clinical failure rate (9 of 418) for aluminous core porcelain crowns and 15.2% (9 of 59) for posterior crowns over a 7-year period. The increased masticatory loading on the central fossae of molar teeth compared with the masticatory forces on anterior crowns was the reason proposed for the increased fracture incidence. Hayashi and coworkers[13] have reported 92% longevity for fired ceramic inlays (G-Cera Cosmotech II, GC, Tokyo, Japan) luted with a resin cement at 6 years, although marginal fracture was detected in 13% of restorations and marginal discoloration in 23%. Fuzzi and Rapelli[14] have reported the survival of 182 ceramic inlays in 66 patients, using Kaplan-Meier statistical analysis to predict a survival rate of 95% at 11.5 years. Thordrup and coworkers[15] assessed Vita Dur (Vita Zahnfabrik, Bad Säckingen, Germany) inlays, cemented with a dual-cure resin cement, at 5 years, finding that 88% were functional.

Glass Infiltration

To further increase the volume of reinforcing alumina crystals, an infiltration technique was employed. In the production of In-Ceram (Vita Zahnfabrik), an alumina body obtained from a slip was fired for 2 hours at 1,125°C to produce a porous, interconnected alumina substructure. Densification of the ceramic was achieved in a second firing at 1,100°C by infiltrating the porous alumina substructure with a low-viscosity lanthanum-based glass. The advantage of In-Ceram was its high strength, reported to be three to four times higher than aluminous core porcelain at 320 to 600 MPa,[7,16–22] combined with low shrinkage that allows exact shaping and a good marginal fit.[23]

Few long-term evaluations of the success of In-Ceram restorations have been reported, but McLaren and White[24] reported a 3-year survival rate of 96% for a sample size of 223 In-Ceram crowns placed in a prosthodontic practice. A variety of luting cements were used in this study, ranging from resin, glass ionomer, resin-modified glass ionomer, and zinc phosphate, with the authors reporting that they used the resin cement routinely but that they used the resin-modified glass ionomer when maximal translucency was required and the phosphate cement for increased opacity.

Castable Glass Ceramics

At room temperature, glass is in a metastable amorphous state that has not crystallized on cooling from the melt. However, controlled crystallization can occur by heating the glass to a suitable, higher temperature in the presence of crystal seeds, or nuclei, to produce a dense mass of tiny interlocking crystals or dispersed crystallites, a process known as *ceramming*.[25] In the 1950s glass ceramics with superior strength were developed by Corning Glass Works in the United States.[26] Industrial development of the cast glass-ceramic system (Dicor Castable Glass Ceramic, Dentsply/York, York, PA) for dental restorations was based on the work of Grossman[27] and Adair.[28] The major components of the glass were silicon dioxide, potassium oxide, magnesium oxide, and magnesium fluoride, along with the minor addition of aluminum oxide and zirconium dioxide for durability. Esthetics were also improved with the addition of a fluorescing agent. The glass-ceramic material retained its amorphous structure throughout the casting process such that the castings were converted to a partially crystalline state by ceramming. Nucleation and growth of mica-type crystals occurring within the body of the material produced a machinable material with enhanced strength and fracture resistance. The intrinsic strength was distributed throughout the body of the castable ceramic restoration since it was formed as a monolithic structure from the interlocking mica crystals.[29] However, surface crystallization did produce a modified structure at fit and exterior surfaces.

Construction of the Dicor crown used the lost-wax process familiar to dental technicians, with the base glass being cast into a mold to produce a glass crown. The glass was cast centrifugally at 1,370°C, producing a crown that was semicrystalline but still translucent. These glass ceramics can only be cast in a single color, but the translucent crown could be colored by surface glazes or thin application of a porcelain veneer.[30] The major advantage of the system was a combination of a lower risk of processing

Table 8-1 Reported success rates of Class I Dicor inlays*

Authors	Observation time	No. of inlays	% fractured	Cement
Stenberg and Matsson[35]	2 y	25	8.9	Glass ionomer
Noack and Roulet[36]	4 y	210	7.6	Resin
Roulet[37]	5 y	116	6.0	Resin
Roulet[38]	6 y	123	5.7	Resin

*After van Dijken et al.[39]

faults, ease of manufacture, excellent fit, and the option for chairside adjustment without significant loss of properties.

Unfortunately, the strength of the Dicor Castable Glass Ceramic was inadequate for the construction of fixed prostheses. A 14-year clinical study to evaluate the survival rate for 1,444 complete-coverage Dicor restorations reported 188 clinical failures resulting in a failure rate of the order of 13%.[31,32] Kelsey and coworkers,[33] following a study of 101 Dicor crowns cemented with a resin cement, reported that 15 of those restorations failed at 4 years and 13 of those failures affected molar teeth. The failure rate was 22.8% in molar teeth and 5.7% in premolar teeth. The authors compared their data with those of Anusavice,[34] who reported a 15.2% failure rate for molar crowns made from aluminous core porcelain and a 6.4% failure rate for premolar restorations. The authors further reported that the majority of the failures occurred after 2 years and surmised that a fatigue-related process is involved. Success rates of Dicor inlays are shown in Table 8-1.

Castable Ceramics

Although a clinically adequate fit was produced with an aluminous core porcelain restoration, shrinkage on firing, distortion of the platinum matrix, and the inherent weakness of dental porcelain limited its effectiveness in clinical dentistry.[40] A carefully constructed all-ceramic porcelain jacket crown has a relatively low flaw content and high strength. On the other hand, commercially manufactured crowns have a higher number of flaws, many of which are introduced during powder condensation of the inner layer, and consequently these crowns have varying strengths.[41] In an attempt to overcome these problems, the Cerestore Non-Shrink Alumina Ceramic (Coors Biomedical, Lakewood, CO) was developed as an alternative reinforcing core material to aluminous core porcelain.[40]

In the Cerestore system, rather than applying the material as a slurry, an inner coping was transfer (injection) molded using the nonshrink alumina-based ceramic. Using the stone die replica of the tooth preparation, a wax model of the re-

119

quired inner coping was built up and used to construct a mold where the core material was then injected when the wax was burnt out.[41] The material achieved high strength from the spinel-based matrix phase but had high levels of porosity after firing, reported by Marquis and Wilson[41] to be up to 20%. Once the inner core had been made, the outer layers were added in the same way as for the aluminous porcelain jacket crown. There is a paucity of reports on the success rates of Cerestore restorations, but Linkowski[42] reported a 4-year failure rate of 18.5% for molar crowns and 3% for anterior crowns, and the material has been withdrawn from the market because of poor performance.[34] Anusavice[34] considers these failure rates to be similar to those of aluminous core jacket crowns.

Pressable Ceramics

The high-strength glass-ceramic IPS Empress (Ivoclar Vivadent, Schaan, Liechtenstein), introduced in 1990, is a leucite (40% to 50%)–reinforced feldspathic porcelain for injection molding.[43] IPS Empress is pre-cerammed so that it has reached its maximum crystallinity prior to processing and does not change after processing, namely after heating in a cylinder form and injection under pressure and high temperature into a mold. The leucite crystals improve the strength, fracture resistance, and resistance to crack propagation of the feldspathic glass matrix in a manner similar to that which occurs in glass ceramics or dispersion-strengthened aluminous porcelains.

A conventional lost-wax technique is used with a special investment material and a prolonged burnout cycle of 90 minutes at 850°C and a heating rate of 3°C/min. The wax patterns are placed in a furnace along with the Empress ingots and heated to approximately 1,200°C. The investment mold is then placed in the bottom of the Empress injection molding system at a temperature of about 1,150°C, and the selected glass ingot is placed in the upper chamber for molding under a pressure close to 0.4 MPa. The ingots are supplied in several shades. Either the restoration is cast to its final contour prior to staining and glazing, or a coping is molded, upon which porcelain is added to achieve the final shape and shade of the restoration.

Fischer et al[44] defined IPS Empress as an all-ceramic material with a glassy matrix embedded with a high proportion (35 vol%) of leucite crystals. The advantages of IPS Empress are that there is no need for metal or an opaque ceramic core, and it has a moderate flexure strength, excellent fit, and esthetics. Its potential to fracture in posterior areas and the need for special laboratory equipment are its major disadvantages. IPS Empress restorations are translucent and have reported flexural strengths of 160 to 180 MPa.[43] Fradeani and Aquilano[45,46] estimated a 95% clinical success rate of 144 anterior and posterior crowns luted with resin cement over 6 to 68 months (mean of 37 months) using the Kaplan-Meier analysis and the modified US Public Health Service criteria. They also conducted a clinical study on 125 posterior IPS Empress inlays over 7 to 56 months (mean of 40.3 months) and estimated a success rate of 96% after 4.5 years.[46] Studer et al[47] conducted a 6-year clinical study of 142 IPS Empress crowns in 59 patients, adhesively cemented (by etching with hydrofluoric acid, silanization,

Table 8-2 Success rates of Empress inlays

Authors	Observation time	No. of inlays	% fractured	Cement
Fradeani and Aquilano[46]	40 mo (mean)	125	4.8	Resin
Molin and Karlsson[48]	5 y	20	20.0	Resin
Studer et al[47]	6 y	163	7.4	Resin
Krämer et al[49]	4 y	96	7.0	Resin
Frankenberger et al[50]	6 y	59	7.0	Resin

application of dentin adhesive, and use of resin cement), that resulted in a success rate of 89%. Other studies reporting the success rates of Empress inlays are presented in Table 8-2. However, although Krämer et al reported a failure rate of 7%, they further reported that 70% of the remaining inlays exhibited marginal deficiencies.[49]

Machinable Ceramics

Machinable ceramics are generally supplied as blocks or ingots in various shades that can be ground into the finished prosthesis without the need for further high-temperature firing. Restorations are constructed by computer-aided design and computer-aided manufacturing (CAD/CAM) or by copy-milling devices, and the restorations are subsequently stained and glazed to achieve the desired esthetic characteristics. Heymann and coworkers[51] have reported no failures among 42 Cerec (Siemens, Bensheim, Germany) inlays luted with resin cement at 4 years.

The Procera (Nobel Biocare, Gothenburg, Sweden) all-ceramic system was introduced by Andersson et al[52,53] and employs high-alumina powders (> 99.9%) to produce densely sintered ceramic copings in the manufacture of all-ceramic crowns. Small amounts of magnesium oxide are added to the alumina powder to facilitate complete sintering.[54] Shrinkage (about 15% to 20%) occurs during sintering of alumina, so that with the development of an enlarging copy-milling machine, enlarged copies of the tooth preparation can be produced to compensate for the shrinkage. The high-purity alumina is pressed on the enlarged die and the outer surface formed using a copy-milling machine that traces the outline of a wax model of the desired restoration. The pressed body is then lifted off the die, trimmed, and sintered to full density. The flexural strength of Procera has been reported to range from 610 to 690 MPa,[55,56] comparable with porcelain-fused-to-metal restorations with negligible porosity.[57]

The process requires the use of elaborate computer and milling machines, which are currently placed at three manufacturing centers owned by the company. Dental dies are not physically shipped to the manufacturer. Instead, they are converted in the dental office or dental laboratory to three-dimensional digital data through scanning (by a contact scanner), and the information is transferred to the manufacturing center electronically via modem and telephone lines. While the imaging equipment is costly and technique sensitive, it allows speedy transfer of die dimensions to the manufacturing centers, which may be remote from the treatment venue. A 5-year clinical study of 100 Procera restorations placed in the anterior and posterior regions of the mouth produced only three crown fractures through the veneering porcelain and alumina coping materials,[58] and the authors concluded that Procera AllCeram crowns may be used in all areas of the mouth. These results are not dissimilar to those reported by Milleding and coworkers[59] for Procera titanium crowns after 2 years, with 3 of 40 crowns placed being unsatisfactory.

The Effect of Adhesive Technology

Laboratory Studies: The Cement Effect

Abdalla and Davidson[60] have reported a laboratory investigation of the marginal integrity of ceramic inlays luted with resin cement, compomer cement, and a conventional glass-ionomer cement. Specimens were subjected to fatigue loading and evaluated for dye penetration. The results indicated significantly better marginal integrity for inlays luted with the resin and compomer luting materials compared with inlays luted with the glass-ionomer material. The authors concluded that ceramic inlays cemented with a resin luting cement demonstrated

increased tolerance to occlusal loading compared with those luted with a glass-ionomer cement.

Mitchell et al[61] tested the fracture toughness of six luting cements (four conventional glass-ionomer cements, one resin-modified glass ionomer, and one resin cement) to determine their likelihood to fail cohesively when loaded. The results indicated that the fracture toughness of the resin-modified glass-ionomer cement was significantly higher than any of the four conventional glass-ionomer cements and that the fracture toughness of the resin composite cement (Scotchbond, 3M Espe, St Paul, MN) was significantly higher than any of the other cements tested. The authors considered that the fracture toughness measurement may provide a more reliable parameter for measuring potential clinical performance than the compressive or diametral tensile strength measurements stipulated in current standards protocols. They further considered that a cement with sufficiently high fracture toughness to prevent cohesive failure under masticatory loading is preferable to one with very high fracture toughness where the weakest link in the restored tooth would be the tensile strength of the dentin.[61]

Knobloch and coworkers[62] have also tested the fracture toughness of luting cements. These workers evaluated three resin composite luting cements, three resin-modified glass-ionomer cements, and a conventional glass-ionomer cement at 24 hours and 7 days. Results indicated that the resin-modified glass-ionomer cements had higher fracture toughness values than the conventional glass-ionomer cement, and that two of

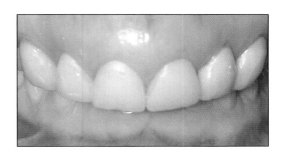

Fig 8-2 Dentin-bonded crowns on the maxillary incisor and canine teeth at 3 years in a patient suffering from erosive tooth substance loss.

the resin cements (C&B Metabond [Parkell, Farmington, NY] and Enforce [Dentsply, Milford, DE]) had higher fracture toughness values than all the other cements, including one of the resin cements tested, Panavia 21 (Kuraray, Osaka, Japan).

Dentin-bonded crowns are becoming more widely used.[63] In these restorations, an all-ceramic crown is luted with a dual-cure resin cement, with the bond being mediated by a dentin bonding agent and the creation of a micromechanically retentive fitting surface by etching the ceramic with hydrofluoric acid.[64] Such restorations have been considered of value in the treatment of patients with tooth substance loss, but they may also be used instead of conventional crowns. There are few long-term evaluations of these restorations, but a retrospective evaluation of 53 crowns at a mean age of 4.4 years has indicated reasonable clinical performance, with 48 (91%) restorations being found to be intact and patient satisfaction levels high.[65] Some dentin-bonded crowns that have been in clinical service for 4 years are shown in Fig 8-2. The advantages of dentin-bonded crowns are:

- The minimal tooth preparation required, which should minimize the risk of an adverse pulpal response
- The excellent esthetics that may be achieved, in part because there is no metal substructure
- The potential for a good gingival response because the margins should be polished smooth and the insoluble resin cement shows no potential for marginal defects
- The potential to treat shortened, worn teeth because the adhesive technique does not demand a preparation with ideal resistance and retention form

Bonding of crowns to stainless steel dies may be considered to be far removed from the clinical situation. However, Groten and Pröbster[66] examined the effect of conditioning the dies by abrading their surfaces with Rocatec (3M Espe) during the compressive loading of 120 Empress crowns. The crowns were cemented to the dies using zinc phosphate cement, a glass-ionomer cement, and a resin cement. Fracture resistance was improved when the fitting surface of the crowns was etched with hydrofluoric acid and sealed with a light-curing bonding agent, but it was optimized when the dies were abraded with Rocatec to implant reactive particles into the metal surface. However, the fracture pattern of the "adhesive" group was more complex than that of the other groups.

Laboratory tests examining fracture resistance of dentin-bonded crowns have been conducted using a standardized preparation, crown manufacture, and placement. These tests have indicated that luting the crown with a dual-cure resin cement, used in conjunction with a dentin bonding agent, produced significantly greater resistance to a compressive force than when zinc phosphate cement is used. Fracture resistance was also decreased when the dentin bonding agent was not used.[67,68] In a related study, no increase in fracture resistance was noted when the occlusal reduction was increased from 2 to 3 mm or when a shoulder rather than a knife-edge preparation was used cervically.[64]

The effect of cement type on the performance of porcelain veneers has seen little testing. Recently, Magne and Douglas[69] used a finite element model to evaluate the extent to which a veneer can mimic the biomechanics of the original tooth. Their results indicated that the placement of a veneer returned the stiffness of a tooth to 96% of its original value, with the treatment restoring both the mechanical behavior and the microstructure of the intact tooth. The reduced fracture resistance when a nonadhesive luting material (zinc phosphate) was used may result from the lack of bonding per se, given that it has been considered that such a cement merely occupies space.[70] It may also result from the poorer physical properties of the

phosphate luting material used, which are comparable with those of other inorganic luting materials but have lower compressive and tensile strengths when compared to resin-based luting materials. However, since this was the luting material of choice for about half a century, it may be construed that its physical properties are adequate for its function.

Other workers have examined the use of conventional cements on fracture resistance of all-ceramic crowns. In a study by Jensen et al,[71] in which a glass-ionomer luting cement was used to lute a group of dentin-bonded all-ceramic crowns, fracture resistance was reduced in comparison to those luted with dentin bonding agents (Scotchbond, 3M Espe, and Gluma, Bayer Dental, Leverkusen, Germany) and a dual-cure resin composite cement. In the cases in which a glass-ionomer cement was used, it might be expected that some bonding would have occurred between dentin and the glass ionomer. However, since fracture resistance was decreased when the glass ionomer was used as luting material, other factors may be involved in the superior fracture resistance of crowns luted with a resin composite–based material. This may partly be explained by the lower bond strengths that were noted between castable ceramic specimens (Dicor) and a glass-ionomer cement as compared to a resin cement.[70] However, the superior fracture resistance may also be explained by the synergistic nature of the bonding together of dentin and porcelain by the intermediary luting cement. Alternatively, the inferior physical properties of the nonresin cements considered above may be involved. These results are similar to those reported by

Dietschi et al,[72] who found that "ceramic inlays cemented with composite resin seemed to resist fracture better than those luted with glass-ionomer, although no statistically significant difference was found."

A further contributory factor has been put forward by Marquis,[73] who considered that the use of a resin-based luting material may reduce the potential for crack propagation by healing surface flaws, thereby producing an enhanced performance when compared with other "conventional" luting materials. He also considered that this might be a factor in the good performance of veneer restorations.

A further explanation for the "strengthening" effect of resin-based luting materials has been proposed by Nathanson.[74] He considered that, while shrinkage during resin composite polymerization is generally viewed as a negative property, within certain limitations, the resin composite polymerization shrinkage may help strengthen porcelain by exerting a force on the inner porcelain surface that stresses porcelain molecules together rather than away from each other. Conversely, it may be conjectured that resin-modified glass-ionomer cements, which have been found to expand on setting under moist conditions, may cause flaws in the ceramic surface to expand and thereby increase the risk of crack propagation. Further research is required to investigate these matters.

Examination of the extent and position of the fractures of specimens in early studies on fracture resistance of dentin-bonded crowns[67,68] showed no difference in the modes of fracture between any of the groups. In all cases, the crown fractured before tooth substance was dam-aged. It therefore appears that while the dentin-bonding procedure may enhance the fracture resistance of all-ceramic crowns, an adhesive luting procedure is not necessarily required to protect underlying tooth structure from fracture. In this respect, work carried out by Jensen et al[71] has demonstrated that resin-bonded, etched porcelain complete-veneer crowns had a fracture resistance approximately equal to that of size-matched natural teeth.

In one of the first papers written on the dentin-bonded crown technique, Crocker[75] compared the fracture resistance of alumina-cored porcelain crowns cemented with zinc phosphate cement with similar crowns cemented with Silux (3M Espe) resin diluted with an unfilled bis-GMA dimethacrylate mixture and Scotchbond 2 dentin adhesive (3M Espe). The details of the experimental procedure were not reported, except that the crowns were "loaded to failure" and that statistical analysis revealed that the crowns luted with resin were "at least as strong" as conventional alumina-cored porcelain crowns. Crocker[75] reported that the mode of fracture of the two types of crown was different, with the crowns luted with resin fracturing as one system and the porcelain acting like an artificial enamel. This finding would appear to be in agreement with that of Grossman,[76] who considered, following photoelastic examination of load-transfer mechanisms, that enhanced clinical performance of bonded glass-ceramic restorations is achieved by transfer of stress through the tooth-crown interface. He demonstrated that the strength of adhesion was significant in reducing stress at the tooth-crown interface.

Recently, polymer crowns without a metal substructure have been suggested as a less expensive alternative to ceramic or metal-ceramic crowns.[77] Rammelsberg and coworkers[78] have examined the fracture resistance of Artglass (Heraeus Kulzer, Wehrheim, Germany) crowns cemented to 72 extracted molar teeth, divided into three groups. Standardized preparations were made, and crowns were constructed and placed using three cements—zinc phosphate, glass ionomer, and resin (2Bond2, Heraeus Kulzer). After thermocycling, a compressive load was applied to failure. None of the 24 crowns placed with zinc phosphate cement had become loose after thermocycling and was recemented prior to testing. The crowns placed using the resin cement failed at significantly greater loads than the crowns placed with the other two cements.

Lastly, in a study by McCormick et al,[79] all-ceramic crowns were luted with zinc phosphate, glass ionomer, or resin composite cements, and results indicated no statistical difference between fracture strengths of the three groups. However, in that study, a dentin-bonding procedure was not carried out with the resin composite group, which may explain the apparent divergence between the results obtained by McCormick et al and those obtained in other studies. It appears that the dentin-bonding procedure is essential if the all-ceramic crown is to be adequately supported by tooth structure.

Laboratory Studies: Surface Strengthening Effects

A number of substrates lead to variations in the fracture resistance of porcelain specimens in laboratory studies. Mesaros and coworkers[80] in a study of 60 beam-shaped Dicor specimens and 40 bovine dentin specimens found that the fracture resistance of the dentin-cement-ceramic complex increased with the intermediate use of a dentin-bonding agent. They concluded that the application of a dentin-bonding agent in conjunction with a dual-cure resin cement may be the system of choice for luting a cast glass-ceramic crown.

Dental cements may be used in practice with a wide range of mixing ratios,[81,82] and as a result, Fleming and Narayan[83] investigated the impact of cement type and mixing on the strength of reinforcing porcelain. The luting agents employed included those advocated for cementing all-ceramic restorations, namely zinc polycarboxylate, conventional glass ionomer, and resin composite cements. Sets of 25 aluminous core porcelain disk specimens were coated with different cement types of varying mixing ratios to produce a luting thickness and stored at 37°C ± 1°C for 24 hours prior to testing. Mean fracture strengths, standard deviations, and associated Weibull moduli (m) were determined using biaxial fracture (ball-on-ring). The plots of survival probability against strength for specimens coated with acid-base cements develop an asymmetry at the lower values of strength. This effect was exacerbated for acid-base cements prepared at mixing ratios below that recommended for luting purposes. Fleming and Narayan[83] concluded that the longevity of all-ceramic crowns prepared in commercial laboratories, which contain strength limiting defects, would be markedly increased if the crowns were luted with resin-based cements, which heal surface flaws, rather than with acid-base cements, which exacerbate flaws by extending them. The corrosive acidic environment of acid-base cements may have extended preexisting flaws in the porcelain disks, producing the asymmetry in the survival distributions. Resin composite cements appeared to enhance the strength of the porcelain disk specimens, possibly by healing the surface imperfections. Fleming and Narayan proposed that this may increase their scope of application over acid-base cements to include the luting of all-ceramic restorations.

Previously, Fleming et al[82] identified that zinc phosphate cements exhibited similar corrosive effects that were more pronounced compared with the acid-base cements employed by Fleming and Narayan.[83] Fleming et al proposed that this was a result of the increased pH of the phosphoric acid liquid component of the zinc phosphate cement, compared with the polyacrylic acid constituent employed in glass-ionomer and polycarboxylate cements. Acid-base cements prepared from powder-liquid mixing ratios below that recommended by the manufacturers have also been shown to extend surface imperfections more than cements manipulated according to the manufacturer's instructions as a result of the increased acidity of the cement mass. It is therefore proposed by the authors[82,83] that to ensure the longevity of all-ceramic restorations in clinical practice non–acid-base cements be employed as the critical step in cementing all-ceramic restorations. Buithieu and Nathanson[84] have investigated the fracture resistance of Dicor ceramic samples placed over or bonded to a base and found that bonding the ceramic to a resin-modified glass-ionomer base produced specimens of greater fracture resistance, as compared with those not bonded and using a conventional glass-ionomer base.

Resin cements therefore appear to have a sealing and/or strengthening effect on ceramic specimens. However, the ceramic surface roughness may also play a part, as was demonstrated by Williamson et al,[85] who in 1996 found that specimens with a coarse ground surface were significantly weaker than those with polished surfaces. Giordano and coworkers[86] have noted that sequential polishing significantly improved the flexural strength of feldspathic porcelain. More recently, a similar effect was demonstrated by de Jager and coworkers.[87] These researchers tested groups of porcelain disks with 12 different finishing procedures. With the exception of one type of ceramic, a significant correlation was found between the specimen surface roughness and the biaxial flexure strength: The smoother the surface, the stronger the specimen.

Clinical Studies: Failure Rates of Conventionally Luted and Adhesively Luted Crowns and Inlays

There are two factors that may occur during the clinical use of adhesive techniques[66]:

• A more effective transfer of stress by the creation of strong bonding forces at the tooth-resin-ceramic interfaces

127

- The strengthening effect resulting from resin coating, following the principles of surface modification to inhibit crack initiation[34]

Despite variations in the fracture strength of the different ceramic materials reported above, the annual clinical failure rate reported for these materials in the dental literature is remarkably consistent.[88,89] These results emphasize that there may be little correlation between the average fracture strength determined by conventional material science techniques and clinical performance. The key failures in all-ceramic systems are those that occur at low levels of applied stress, since even with the relatively weaker systems a failure rate of 50% (which relates to the average fracture strength) will not occur for more than 15 years. If ceramics are to be used for dental applications, then more detailed information on the statistical variations in strength is clearly required. Perhaps the conventional cements used with many crowns in the past have not provided the necessary transfer of stress from restoration to tooth.

The restoration of function and esthetics of the coronal part of the tooth (preferably without causing damage to the pulp) is by far the most common indication for the use of all-ceramic crowns in the restoration of anterior teeth. However, all-ceramic restorations consist of a layer of ceramic between 1.0- and 2.0-mm thick. As a result of this tooth reduction, there is potential for pulpal irritation, especially if the dentinal tubules are left exposed rather than sealed. The use of a conventional acid-base luting material such as zinc phosphate, which has no inherent

ability to seal dentin and prevent microleakage, may also potentiate the occurrence of pulp problems. Furthermore, the crown will be held in contact with the supporting thickness of dentin through a layer of cement 30 to 100 µm thick. Consequently, ceramic restorations are uniformly supported on a relatively elastic foundation that is not easily reproduced by laboratory load-to-failure mechanical tests. Previous investigations,[31,32,73,89] however, have identified higher survival rates for all-ceramic crowns cemented and bonded with resin composite cements compared with acid-base (zinc phosphate and glass ionomer) cements. The elimination or blunting of flaws on the inner surface of the restoration was the proposed strengthening effect that led to the increased longevity associated with resin cements.[90] However, hydroscopic expansion of some resin composite cements has led to post-cementation fracture of all-ceramic crowns when these materials were employed as adhesive luting agents.[91,92] As a result, an investigation into the potential for increased longevity of these resin composite cements needs to be established to identify if porcelain needs to be supported or not.

A number of authors have compared the success rates of restorations luted with conventional (that is, acid-base) luting materials and those luted with resin-based luting materials and using adhesive procedures, which include the use of a dentin-bonding agent, a micromechanically retentive ceramic fitting surface, and the application of a silane to promote the adhesion of the ceramic to the resin-based luting material. However, there are lamentably few long-term evaluations of the success rates of ceramic restorations.

Malament and Socransky[31,32] assessed the survival of 1,444 Dicor crowns in 417 patients in a private practice for up to 14 years. Crowns were placed using zinc phosphate, glass-ionomer, or various types of resin cement. A total of 180 failures were recorded (12.5%, or 2.5% per year). These workers found that etching of the fitting surface improved the success rate, with survival of etched restorations being 74% at 14 years and that of nonetched restorations being 54%. Van Dijken and coworkers[93] assessed the clinical performance of 118 fired ceramic inlays (Mirage Chameleon Dental Products, Kansas City, KS) placed in Class II cavities in premolar and molar teeth. At 6 years, 12.1% of the restorations that were luted with resin composite and enamel bonding were considered unacceptable because of partial fracture, postoperative sensitivity, secondary caries, and large marginal defects. Dentin-bonding procedures were not used. In the group of inlays luted with glass-ionomer cement, 26.3% of the restorations were deemed unacceptable because of total loss, partial fracture, and secondary caries. The bonding failures occurred mostly between the ceramic inlay and the glass-ionomer cement. In their discussion of the results, van Dijken et al[93] stated that "the adhesion of the glass-ionomer cement to etched porcelain is inferior to that achieved with micromechanical bonding of resin composite luting agents." It is worth noting that none of the adhesively luted inlays were lost by a total debond, while this was the most prevalent reason for the loss of the inlays cemented with glass ionomer.[93] A 3-year evaluation of these fired ceramic inlays showed that 15.3% of the inlays luted with glass ionomer were unacceptable, compared with 3.4% of those in the resin composite group.[94] Con-

versely, Sjögren and coworkers[95] assessed Dicor crowns in practice at a mean age of 6.1 years. Of the 98 crowns examined, 82% were rated satisfactory. However, the authors found no difference in the success rates of crowns cemented with glass-ionomer, phosphate, or resin cements.

Results of studies of castable glass-ceramic (Dicor) inlays luted with a resin cement have indicated a failure rate of 13% after 4 years.[36] However, in a study in which the Dicor inlays were luted with a glass-ionomer cement, the failure rate was 23% after 5 years.[35] With regard to feldspathic porcelain, Isidor and Brondum[96] reported a failure rate of 80% when they assessed 10 porcelain inlays luted with light-cured resin cement, after a mean of 40 months. The same authors reported that 2 similar inlays (of 11) luted with a dual-cure resin cement failed between 20 and 39 months. The authors attributed the high failure rate to a less-than-ideal thickness of ceramic and to the inadequate cure of the light-cure resin cement where the porcelain inlay was thickest.

As stated previously, Kelsey and coworkers[33] reported a study of 101 Dicor crowns cemented with a resin cement, with a failure rate of 22.8% in molar teeth and 5.7% in premolar teeth. These data may be compared with those from Moffa et al,[97] who reported a failure rate of 35% for Dicor crowns cemented with zinc phosphate cement.

Concluding Remarks

From the foregoing, there would appear to be evidence from clinical studies that crowns luted with a resin cement and with the placement procedure incorporating dentin bonding have enhanced rates of survival. Laboratory studies also confirm the enhanced resistance to fracture of crowns cemented with an adhesive procedure. However, the "crunch the crown" methodology of some laboratory studies examining fracture resistance of all-ceramic crowns has been criticized by Kelly,[98] who quoted seven papers in which the loads to failure were "extremely high" (1,500 to 5,000 N) compared with those measured during mastication and swallowing. Nevertheless, the laboratory data indicates improved laboratory performance when adhesive techniques are employed. Kelly further stated that traditional tests cause modes of failure that produce many fragments.[98] In the articles cited above, the crowns did not produce a large number of fragments on fracturing, but instead the compressive forces caused a crack in the crown without a debond; in other words, a "segment" of the crown fractured and debonded in a manner similar to that seen in the clinical situation. Furthermore, a majority of the sources quoted above have employed techniques in the laboratory that replicate those in the clinic. Laboratory data should always be extrapolated with caution to the clinical situation, but the previously mentioned studies may at least allow comparison between groups (such as those with and without the use of a dentin-bonding agent). However, the ability of resin to seal flaws in ceramic surfaces seems unchallenged by Kelly's research.

Therefore, the use of resin as a luting material for ceramic restorations is strongly suggested, given that research

from three different aspects—laboratory fracture studies comparing restorations luted with resin versus other materials and both clinical and laboratory studies examining the surface sealing/strengthening effect of resin on ceramic—indicates the beneficial effect of resin.

References

1. Weinstein M, Katz S, Weinstein AB [inventors]. Permanent Manufacturing Corp, assignee. Fused porcelain-to-metal teeth. US patent 3,052,982. 11 Sept 1962.

2. Brune D. Metal release from dental biomaterials. Biomaterials 1986;7:163–175.

3. Land CH. Porcelain dental art. Dent Cosmos 1903;45:437–444.

4. Land CH. Porcelain dental art, No. 2. Dent Cosmos 1903;45:615–620.

5. Clark EB. Requirements of the jacket crown. J Am Dent Assoc 1939;26:355–363.

6. McLean JW. The strengthening of dental porcelain. In: The Science and Art of Dental Ceramics. Vol I: The Nature of Dental Ceramics and Their Clinical Use, monograph II. Chicago: Quintessence, 1979:55–114.

7. White SN, Caputo AA, Vidjak FMA, Seghi RR. Moduli of rupture of layered dental ceramics. Dent Mater 1994;10:52–58.

8. McLean JW. The nature of dental ceramics. In: The Science and Art of Dental Ceramics. Vol I: The Nature of Dental Ceramics and Their Clinical Use, monograph I. Chicago: Quintessence, 1979:23–51.

9. Binns DB. The testing of alumina ceramics for engineering applications. J Br Ceram Soc 1965;2:294–308.

10. McLean JW, Hughes TH. The reinforcement of dental porcelain with ceramic oxides. Br Dent J 1965;119:251–267.

11. Austin CR, Schofield HZ, Haldy NL. Alumina whiteware. J Am Ceram Soc 1946;29:341–349.

12. McLean JW. The Development of Ceramic Oxide–Reinforced Dental Porcelains with an Appraisal of Their Physical and Chemical Properties [thesis]. London: University of London, 1966.

13. Hayashi M, Tsuchitani Y, Miura M, Takeshige F, Ebisu S. Six-year clinical evaluation of fired ceramic inlays. Oper Dent 1998;23:318–326.

14. Fuzzi M, Rappelli G. Ceramic inlays: Clinical assessment and survival rate. J Adhes Dent 1999;1:71–79.

15. Thordrup M, Isidor F, Horsted-Binslev P. A 5-year clinical study of indirect and direct resin composite and ceramic inlays. Quintessence Int 2001;32:199–205.

16. Claus H. Vita In-Ceram: A new system for producing aluminum oxide crown and bridge substructures. Quintessenz Zahntech 1990;16:35–46.

17. Levy H. Working with the In-Ceram Porcelain System [in French]. Prosth Dent 1990;44:1–11.

18. Marquis PM, Fisher SE. The critical role of surfaces in limiting the performance of dental ceramics [abstract 1272]. J Dent Res 1993;72:262.

19. Sorensen JA, Avera SP, Fanuscu MI. Effect of veneer porcelain on all-ceramic crown strength [abstract 1718]. J Dent Res 1992;71:320.

20. Sorensen JA, Choi C, Fanuscu MI, Mito WT. IPS Empress crown system: Three-year clinical trial results. J Calif Dent Assoc 1998;26:130–136.

21. Pröbster L, Diehl J. Slip-casting alumina ceramics for crown and bridge restorations. Quintessence Int 1992;23:25–31.

22. Kappert HF, Knode H. In-Ceram: Testing a new ceramic material. Quintessence Dent Technol 1993;16:87–97.

23. Hornberger H. Strength Microstructure Relationships in a Dental Alumina Glass Composite [thesis]. Birmingham, UK: University of Birmingham, 1995.

24. McLaren EA, White SN. Survival of In-Ceram crowns in a private practice: A prospective clinical trial. J Prosthet Dent 2000;83:216–222.

25. MacCulloch WT. Advances in dental ceramics. Br Dent J 1968;124:361–365.

26. Corning develops new ceramic material. Am Ceram Soc Bull 1957;36:279–280.

27. Grossman DG. Machinable glass-ceramics based on tetrasilicic mica. J Am Ceram Soc 1972;55:446–449.

28. Adair PJ [inventor]. Dental products and processes involving mica compositions. US patent 4,431,420. 14 Feb 1984.

29. Grossman DG, Adair PJ. The castable ceramic crown. Int J Periodontics Restorative Dent 1984;4:33–45.

30. McLean JW. Ceramics in clinical dentistry. Br Dent J 1988;164:187–194.

31. Malament KA, Socransky SS. Survival of Dicor glass-ceramic dental restorations over 14 years: Part I. Survival of Dicor complete coverage restorations and effect of internal surface acid etching, tooth position, gender, and age. J Prosthet Dent 1999;81:23–32.

32. Malament KA, Socransky SS. Survival of Dicor glass-ceramic dental restorations over 14 years: Part II. Effect of thickness of Dicor material and design of tooth preparation. J Prosthet Dent 1999;81:662–667.

33. Kelsey WP, Cavel WT, Blankenau RJ, Barkmeier WW, Wildwerding TM, Latta MA. Four-year study of castable ceramic crowns. Am J Dent 1995;8:259–262.

34. Anusavice KJ. Recent developments in restorative dental ceramics. J Am Dent Assoc 1993;124:72–84.

35. Stenberg R, Matsson L. Clinical evaluation of glass ceramic inlays (Dicor). Acta Odontol Scand 1993;51:91–97.

36. Noack MJ, Roulet JF. Survival rates and mode of failure of Dicor inlays after 4 years [abstract 759]. J Dent Res 1994;73:196.

37. Roulet JF. The longevity of glass ceramic inlays [abstract 36]. J Dent Res 1995;74:425.

38. Roulet JF. Longevity of glass ceramic inlays and amalgam—Results up to 6 years. Clin Oral Invest 1997;1:40–46.

39. Van Dijken JWV, Ormin A, Olofsson A-L. Clinical performance of pressed ceramic inlays luted with resin-modified glass ionomer and autopolymerizing resin composite cements. J Prosthet Dent 1999;82:529–535.

40. Sozio RB, Riley EJ. Esthetic considerations of the all-ceramic crown. J Can Dent Assoc 1984;12:117–121.

41. Marquis PM, Wilson HJ. A tooth for a tooth—Ceramics in modern dentistry. Chem Ind 1986:657–661.

42. Linkowski G. Langzeituntersuchung bei Einem Vollkeramik-Knonensystem (Cerestore) [thesis]. Zurich, Switzerland: University of Zurich, 1989.

43. Gorman CM, McDevitt WE, Hill RG. Comparison of two heat-pressed all-ceramic dental materials. Dent Mater 2000;6:389–395.

44. Fischer H, Maier HR, Marx R. Improved reliability of leucite-reinforced glass by ion exchange. Dent Mater 2000;16:120–128.

45. Fradeani M, Aquilano A. Longitudinal study of pressed glass-ceramic inlays for four and a half years. J Prosthet Dent 1997;78:346–353.

46. Fradeani M, Aquilano A. Clinical experience with Empress crowns. Int J Prosthodont 1997; 10:241–247.

47. Studer S, Lehner C, Brodbeck U, Schärer P. Six-year results of leucite-reinforced glass ceramic crowns. Acta Med Dent Helv 1998;3:218–225.

48. Molin MK, Karlsson SL. A randomized 5-year clinical evaluation of 3 ceramic inlay systems. Int J Prosthodont 2000;13:194–200.

49. Krämer N, Frankenberger R, Pelka M, Petscheldt A. IPS Empress inlays and onlays after four years—A clinical study. J Dent 1999; 27:325–331.

50. Frankenberger R, Petscheldt A, Krämer N. Leucite-reinforced glass ceramic inlays and onlays after 6 years: Clinical behavior. Oper Dent 2000;25:459–465.

51. Heymann HO, Bayne SC, Sturdevant JR, Wilder AD, Robertson TM. The clinical performance of CAD-CAM–generated ceramic inlays. J Am Dent Assoc 1996;127:1171–1181.

52. Andersson M, Oden A. A new all-ceramic crown. Acta Odontol Scand 1993;51:59–64.

53. Andersson M, Razzoog ME, Oden A, Hegenbarth EA, Lang BR. Procera: A new way to achieve an all-ceramic crown. Quintessence Int 1998;29:285–296.

54. Cahoon HP, Christensen CJ. Sintering and grain growth of alumina. J Am Ceram Soc 1956;39: 337–344.

55. Wagner WC, Chu TM. Bi-axial flexure strength and indentation fracture toughness of three new dental core ceramics. J Prosthet Dent 1996;76:140–144.

56. Zeng K, Oden A, Rowcliffe D. Flexure tests on dental ceramics. Int J Prosthodont 1996;9:434–449.

57. May KB, Russell MM, Razzoog ME, Lang BR. Precision of fit: The Procera AllCeram crown. J Prosthet Dent 1998;80:394–404.

58. Oden A, Andersson M, Krystek-Ondracek I, Magnusson D. Five-year clinical evaluation of Procera AllCeram crowns. J Prosthet Dent 1998;80:450–456.

59. Milleding P, Haag P, Neroth B, Renz I. Two years of clinical experience with Procera titanium crowns. Int J Prosthodont 1998;11:224–232.

60. Abdalla AI, Davidson CL. Marginal integrity after fatigue loading of ceramic inlay restorations luted with three different cements. Am J Dent 2000;13:77–80.

61. Mitchell CA, Douglas WH, Cheng Y-S. Fracture toughness of conventional, resin-modified glass-ionomer and composite luting cements. Dent Mater 1999;15:7–13.

62. Knobloch LA, Kerby RE, Seghi R, Berlin JS, Lee JS. Fracture toughness of resin-based luting cements. J Prosthet Dent 2000;83:204–209.

63. Christensen GJ. Should we be bonding all tooth restorations? J Am Dent Assoc 1994;125: 193–194.

64. Burke FJT. Fracture resistance of teeth restored with dentin-bonded crowns: The effect of increased tooth preparation. Quintessence Int 1996;27:115–121.

65. Burke FJT, Qualtrough AJE. Follow-up evaluation of a series of dentin-bonded ceramic restorations. J Esthet Dent 2000;12:16–22.

66. Groten M, Pröbster L. The influence of different cementation modes on the fracture resistance of feldspathic ceramic crowns. Int J Prosthodont 1997;10:169–177.

67. Burke FJT, Watts DC. Fracture resistance of teeth restored with dentin-bonded crowns. Quintessence Int 1994;25:335–340.

68. Burke FJT. The effect of variations in bonding procedure on fracture resistance of dentin-bonded crowns. Quintessence Int 1995;26:293–300.

69. Magne P, Douglas WH. Porcelain veneers: Dentin bonding optimization and biomimetic recovery of the crown. Int J Prosthodont 1999; 12:111–121.

70. Innes-Ledoux PM, Ledoux WR, Weinberg R. A bond strength study of luted castable ceramic restorations. J Dent Res 1989;68:823–825.

71. Jensen ME, Sheth JJ, Tolliver D. Etched-porcelain resin-bonded full-veneer crowns. In vitro fracture resistance. Compend Contin Dent Educ 1989;10:336–347.

72. Dietschi D, Maeder M, Meyer J-M, Holz J. In vitro resistance to fracture of porcelain inlays bonded to tooth. Quintessence Int 1990;21:823–831.

73. Marquis PM. The influence of cements on the mechanical performance of dental ceramics. In: Proceedings of the Fifth International Symposium on Ceramics in Medicine, vol 5, Bioceramics. Japan: Kobunshi Kankokai, 1992:317–324.

74. Nathanson D. Principles of porcelain use as an inlay/onlay material. In: Garber DA, Goldstein RE (eds). Porcelain and Composite Inlays and Onlays. Chicago: Quintessence, 1994:22–25.

75. Crocker WP. The cementation of porcelain jacket crowns with adhesive resins. Br Dent J 1992;172:64–67.

76. Grossman DG. Photoelastic examination of bonded crown interfaces [abstract 719]. J Dent Res 1989;68:271.

77. Clinical Research Associates. Filled polymer crowns—1- and 2-year status reports. CRA Newsletter 1998;22:1–3.

78. Rammelsberg P, Eickemeyer G, Erdelt K, Pospiech P. Fracture resistance of posterior metal-free polymer crowns. J Prosthet Dent 2000;84:303–308.

79. McCormick JT, Rowland W, Shillingburg HT, Duncanson MG. Effect of luting media on the compressive strengths of two types of all-ceramic crown. Quintessence Int 1993;24:405–408.

80. Mesaros AJ, Evans DB, Schwartz RS. Influence of a dentin bonding agent on the fracture load of Dicor. Am J Dent 1994;7:137–140.

81. Fleming GJP, Shelton RM, Marquis PM. The influence of clinically induced variability on the biaxial fracture strength of aluminous core porcelain discs. J Dent 1999;27:587–594.

82. Fleming GJP, Shelton RM, Marquis PM. The influence of clinically induced variability on the biaxial fracture strength of cemented aluminous core porcelain discs. Dent Mater 1999;15:62–70.

83. Fleming GJP, Narayan O. The effect of cement type and mixing on the bi-axial fracture strength of cemented aluminous core porcelain discs. Dent Mater 2003;19:69–76.

84. Buithieu H, Nathanson D. Effect of ionomer base on ceramic resistance to fracture [abstract 572]. J Dent Res 1993;72:175.

85. Williamson RT, Kovarik RE, Mitchell RJ. Effects of grinding, polishing, and overglazing on the flexural strength of a high-leucite feldspathic porcelain. Int J Prosthodont 1996;9:30–37.

86. Giordano RA, Campbell S, Pober R. Flexural strength of feldspathic porcelain treated with ion exchange, overglaze and polishing. J Prosthet Dent 1994;71:468–472.

87. de Jager N, Feilzer AJ, Davidson CL. The influence of surface roughness on porcelain strength. Dent Mater 2000;16:381–388.

88. Miller A, Long J, Miller B, Cole J. Comparison of the fracture strengths of ceramometal crowns versus several all-ceramic crowns. J Prosthet Dent 1992;68:38–41.

89. Rosenstiel SF, Gupta PK, van der Sluys RA, Zimmerman MH. Strength of a dental glass-ceramic after surface coating. Dent Mater 1993;9:274–279.

90. Kelly JR, Nishimura I, Campbell SD. Ceramics in dentistry: Historical roots and current perspectives. J Prosthet Dent 1996;75:18–32.

91. Leevailoj C, Platt JA, Cochran MA, Moore BK. In vitro study of fracture incidence and compressive fracture load of all-ceramic crowns cemented with resin-modified glass ionomer and other luting agents. J Prosthet Dent 1998;80:699–707.

92. Sindel J, Frankenberger R, Krämer N, Petschelt A. Crack formation of all-ceramic crowns dependent on different core build-up and luting materials. J Dent 1999;27:175–181.

93. Van Dijken JWV, Hoglund-Aberg C, Olofsson A-L. Fired ceramic inlays: A 6-year follow-up. J Dent 1998;26:219–225.

94. Hoglund-Aberg C, van Dijken JWV, Olofsson A-L. Three-year comparison of fired ceramic inlays cemented with composite resin or glass-ionomer cement. Acta Odontol Scand 1994;52:140–149.

95. Sjögren G, Lanitto R, Tillberg A. Clinical evaluation of all-ceramic crowns (Dicor) in general practice. J Prosthet Dent 1999;8:177–284.

96. Isidor F, Brondum K. A clinical evaluation of porcelain inlays. J Prosthet Dent 1995;74:140–144.

97. Moffa JP, Lugassey AA, Ellison JA. Clinical evaluation of a castable ceramic material [abstract 43]. J Dent Res 1988;67:118.

98. Kelly JR. Clinically relevant approach to failure testing of all-ceramic retorations. J Prosthet Dent 1999;81:652–661.

Chapter 9

Ceramic Inlays Cemented Adhesively with Glass-Ionomer Cement and Resin Composite Luting Agents

Jan W. V. van Dijken

Abstract

This chapter reviews different ceramics and the influence of luting agents on the durability of ceramic inlays and onlays. The dental literature was reviewed for longitudinal, controlled clinical studies of ceramic inlays and onlays luted with different luting agents. Longevity and annual failure were determined. Phosphate cements, light-cured resin composites, and conventional glass-ionomer cements showed unacceptable, high clinical failure rates and are not suitable for luting dental ceramic inlays. Dual-cured and chemically cured resin composites and a resin-modified glass-ionomer cement showed better durability. Inlays of pressed ceramics and computer-aided design/computer assisted manufacture (CAD/CAM)–produced ceramics showed better longevity than fired-ceramic inlays.

The popularity of tooth-colored posterior restorations has increased due to demand for esthetic restoratives and also a growing concern about the biocompatibility of amalgam. Posterior composites have been used increasingly during the last years. Despite promising results, polymerization shrinkage, surface wear in contact areas, and a growing concern about biocompatibility and leakage of components of aged resin composite have been named as disadvantages.

Ceramics possess many characteristics that make them desirable for dental restorative materials. They are considered the most biocompatible of all dental materials, are less subject to chemical degradation than other dental materials, and are able to reproduce the natural appearance of the tooth.[1] Unfortunately, they tend to be brittle and fracture with little or no permanent deformation.[2] Although direct-fired all-ceramic restorations have been advocated for many

135

years, interest in porcelain revived after the introduction of stronger ceramics and because of the fact that most all-ceramic materials can be etched with hydrofluoric acid or ammonium bifluoride and bonded to the underlying conditioned tooth structures.[3] The increased surface roughness of enamel, dentin, and ceramic surfaces promotes mechanical interlocking of the resin composite luting agent to these surfaces.[4] A silane treatment is thought to contribute to covalent bond formation between the ceramic surface and the composite, and it also improves wetting of the ceramic surface by the resin composite cement. The concept of bonding ceramics to tooth substance has been applied to the manufacture of veneers, inlays, onlays, and partial and full-coverage restorations. The improved bonding has led to change away from traditional methods of preparation for retention and resistance forms necessary for conventional cements.[5]

Ceramics

Ceramics are defined as nonmetallic and inorganic materials formed after baking at high temperatures.[6] They contain fabrication defects created during processing and/or cracks induced by machining or grinding.[7,8] Porosities and cracks have been shown to be fracture initiation sites. Over the past years these limitations have been addressed with several approaches to strengthen these materials. Early ceramics were amorphous in structure and very weak. Crystalline structures are generally stronger because their atoms are in a state of maximum packing density. Increasing the crystalline content

of conventional feldspathic porcelain developed stronger all-ceramic systems. All of these systems used the refractory die technique. In this technique, the porcelain is built up in layers, with a powder-water slurry, on a model. The layering technique gives a less-controlled crystallization. Dental ceramics contain a glassy matrix reinforced by various crystalline phases, such as leucite (a potassium aluminosilicate), alumina, or mica. Leucite-reinforced feldspathic ceramics are stronger than conventional feldspathic porcelain.[3,9]

Castable Ceramics

The disadvantage of all these systems is that when the particles are sintered together, microporosities and inhomogeneities can develop between the particles and lead to crack formation. Dicor (Dentsply, Konstanz, Germany) is a mica-based glass-ceramic that is initially made as a glass by the lost-wax technique and centrifugal casting. This is followed by preparing the glass-ceramic by controlled crystallization in a special heat process called *ceramming*. The glass is subsequently converted into a stronger crystalline body, which enhances the strength. Layers of conventional feldspathic shade porcelain then cover the cerammed restoration.

Heat-Pressed, Injection-Molded Ceramics

To overcome the processing of inhomogeneities and porosities during ceramming, a heat-process technique has been developed by the manufacturer using a preccerammed material, also called in-gots. With IPS Empress (Ivoclar Vivadent, Schaan, Liechtenstein), leucite-reinforced feldspathic ceramic ingots are heated and pressed into a refractory mold made by the lost-wax technique (heat press-ing). Additional firing results in a 40% vol-ume of leucite crystals, which signifi-cantly improves the flexural strength. Staining or veneering obtains the final color.[10] According to the manufacturer, IPS Empress II material consists of a lithium disilicate glass-ceramic as the core material with three times greater mechanical properties than the conven-tional Empress. A sintered glass-ceramic that also exhibits a crystalline content is used for veneering.

Infiltrated Ceramics

The use of high-strength ceramic cores has recently led to further development of the slip-casting technique, in which a solid layer is built up on the surface of a porous mold that absorbs the liquid phase by means of capillary forces. Glass-infiltrated alumina is a promising dental ceramic because of its reported strength and toughness. A high-strength alumina coping was introduced as In-Ceram (Vita Zahnfabrik, Bad Säckingen, Germany). The method involves a process called *melt infiltration*, in which a special glass is infiltrated into a preform (the first form of the inlay/crown core) of fused alumina particles. The infiltrated ceramics have the highest fracture toughness and flexural strength, and the hardness of the materials makes it unsuit-able for acid etching with hydrofluoric acid. The core is coated with feldspathic porcelain to enhance esthetics.

Luting Agents

Dental materials that effectively adhere to tooth structure can substantially improve restorative dentistry. Good marginal adaptation between the restorative mate-rial and the cavity walls is essential for prevention of microleakage and retention of the restoration, factors that are often the most important for clinical success. *Adhesion* can be defined as the attraction exhibited between the molecules of dif-ferent materials at their interface. The cri-teria for adhesion to be achieved include a clean substrate for intimate access of adhesive to its surface, complete wetting of the substrate surface, and liquid-to-solid transformation of the adhesive.

The cementation of indirect restora-tions has become more complex in re-cent years. The traditional zinc phos-phate cement used for decades to lute traditional metal crowns can be replaced in many clinical cases by new types of lut-ing agents. The selection of one luting agent over another can be complex and involve a number of parameters such as handling characteristics, physical and mechanical properties, number of shades, ease of removing excess mate-rial, radiopacity, anticariogenic proper-ties, dissolution over time, and adhesion.

Zinc Phosphate Cements

The traditional zinc phosphate cement is based on zinc oxide, magnesium oxide, and other metal oxides mixed in an aqueous solution of phosphoric acid buffered by aluminum and zinc salts. The mixing of zinc phosphate cement is tech-nique sensitive. The aim is to incorporate as much powder into the liquid as possible, while still maintaining as low a film thickness as possible. Cavity varnish has been used to decrease postoperative sensitivity after cementation, but the hydrophobic varnish decreased the wetting of the cement as well as adaptation and retention.[11] Zinc phosphate cements have shown an acceptable seating, strength, and solubility in patients with low caries risk. They are, however, inferior to glass-ionomer cements concerning solubility, bonding to tooth substance, and strength. The cement enjoyed clinical popularity for many years but showed a considerable dissolution in situ and had no adhesion or cariostatic properties. The main cause of failure of traditional fixed partial dentures was secondary caries, which accounted for 30% to 40% of the failures.[12] Loss of retention was the second cause of failure, indicating the importance of correct crown preparation with optimal length, minimal taper, and presence of a cylinder of parallelism. Deficient marginal adaptation and periodontal problems accounted for a further 11% of failures.

Polycarboxylate Cements

Polycarboxylate cements are formed by mixing an aqueous solution of polyacrylic acid and other carboxylic acids, with zinc oxide, magnesium oxide, and alumina or other salts. The film thickness and strength are comparable to those of zinc phosphate cement, but they have a high solubility. The cements have been suggested to adhere chemically to tooth substance. Their initial popularity decreased quickly due to the limitations of the cement.

Glass-Ionomer Cements

Glass-ionomer luting cements are acid-base cements based on the reaction of various polyacrylic acids, copolymers of acrylic, itaconic, tartaric, and maleic acids as well as calcium fluoroalumino glasses. After setting, the cement releases fluoride. The set glass-ionomer luting cements have a lower solubility, higher strength, better radiopacity, and higher fluoride releases than zinc phosphate cements. In addition, the improved adhesion between glass-ionomer cement and tooth substance decreased marginal leakage and increased retention, as compared with zinc phosphate cement. Excess cement has to be removed immediately, and the margins have to be protected from water or saliva during the initial setting phase. Glass-ionomer cements are hydrophilic, and desiccation of dentin before luting can result in postoperative sensitivity. Correctly handled, the use of glass-ionomer cement results in lower postoperative sensitivity than when zinc phosphate cements are used.[13]

An 8-year retrospective study of 1,435 cast crowns showed favorable durability of the cement with a low rate of secondary caries and excellent retention. Of 1,184 vital teeth, 2.4% required subsequent endodontic treatment.[14] Postoperative sensitivity was observed in 3.1%.

Resin-Modified Glass-Ionomer Cements

Resin-modified glass-ionomer cements (RMGICs) are a hybrid version of glass-ionomer cements that contain resin components. The actual formulations of the commercial cements vary considerably.

They contain a glass-ionomer calcium aluminosilicate glass and polyacrylic acid, which undergo an acid-base reaction to form a polysalt hydrogel. Hydroxyethyl methacrylate (HEMA) is added to the resin in most cements, while in some materials the polyacrylic acid is modified with a backbone of pendant polymerizable methacrylate chains. The restorative materials can be light cured, while the luting agents are self-cured. The properties of RMGICs fall between those of conventional glass-ionomer cements and resin composites. The modified cements are stronger and less sensitive to desiccation and early moisture contamination compared with the conventional cements, but show equal fluoride release and adhesion. The RMGICs have been available as a restorative material since the early 1990s and have performed well in nonloaded situations.[15]

The manufacturer of one RMGIC suggests the use of a dentin conditioner, which is composed of 10% citric acid, 2% ferric chloride, and water; another manufacturer recommends the use of a dentin-bonding agent as pretreatment. Few cases of postoperative sensitivity have been reported with the use of RMGIC. The auto-cured luting versions polymerize more slowly and demonstrate greater stress relief and fewer shrinkage effects from the resin part of the cement.

Resin-modified cements have a significant expansion as a result of water sorption. Excessive expansion was a clinical problem for one of the first cements marketed as a lining material, due to its high concentration of HEMA. Several anecdotal reports have stated the expansion of RMGIC luting agents has caused frac-tures in all-ceramic crowns. Cracking of all-ceramic crowns was reported in vitro when one RMGIC (Advance, Caulk/ Dentsply, Milford, DE) was used as a luting agent.[16] It was concluded that the water sorption of the cement resulted in an expansion sufficient to fracture the ceramic restoration. According to the authors, Advance cement should not be classified as an RMGIC because polyacids in the material had been replaced with polymerizable monomers or prepolymers that did not support an acid-base reaction. This material has been withdrawn from the market. Leevailoj et al[17] evaluated the fracture incidence of porcelain jacket all-ceramic crowns cemented with five luting agents, including Advance and two RMGIC luting agents. For the cements studied, only crowns cemented with Advance demonstrated fracture during 2-month storage.

Resin Composites

Resin composites were introduced as restorative materials during the early 1960s but received acceptance as luting agents no earlier than the 1990s. The newer resin composites are highly filled materials with inorganic glass fillers based on improved cross-linked polymers formulated from bisphenol glycidyl methacrylate (bis-GMA) or urethane dimethacrylate (UDMA) resins. The cements are generally modified restorative resin composites that, when combined with a good bonding system, can provide a strong, retentive, and sealed luting interface.[18] Reduction of filler particle size and addition of diluent monomers have overcome initial problems with film thickness. Current dentin-bonding agents used with resin composite cements are strong enough to maintain a bond to tooth structure despite the forces of polymerization shrinkage.[19–21] Excess set resin cement in inaccessible proximal cervical locations can be difficult to remove and should be avoided by careful removal before setting.[22]

Resin composite luting agents are available in chemically cured, light-cured, and dual-cured formulations. The chemically cured cements have the drawback of limited working time and prolonged setting time. Light-cured resin cements have been used for cementation of veneers. Decreased curing depth with increased thickness of the inlay caused by light attenuation has limited their use to laminate veneers.

Self-cured (or chemically cured) two-part materials, involving base and catalyst components, are not light sensitive and polymerize only by chemical reaction. A highly retentive self-cured cement is Panavia 21, a revised formulation of Panavia Ex (Kuraray, Osaka, Japan), which was a powder-liquid material. The cement is effective for clinical bonding to nonprecious metals and ceramics. However, it is technique sensitive and sets extremely quickly under anaerobic conditions. It has a thin film thickness, is several times stronger than zinc phosphate, reduces microleakage, and increases retention.[23] A good bond to ceramic interfaces, which cannot be treated with hydrofluoric acid like In-Ceram and AllCeram (Nobel Biocare, Gothenburg, Sweden), can be achieved with Panavia.[3]

In deeper parts of the cavity, light intensity is too low or absent to polymerize light-cured materials. To ensure optimal conversion, a self-cure or chemical initiator-activator system is combined with the visible light photo initiation system in the so-called dual-cured materials. The cement is exposed to a light source, mostly indirectly, resulting in attenuation of light intensity by overlying tooth tissue, resin composite, or ceramic material. Watts and Cash[24] reported that the reflection of visible blue light from the surfaces of natural and synthetic ceramics and composite dental biomaterials is in the range of 30% to 90%, depending on the material. There is a high degree of inefficiency in the transmission of the visible light into and through esthetic biomaterials. A self-cure peroxide/amine or equivalent system is present to produce free radicals and polymerization at depths in the cement not reached by sufficient light. Ideally, the self-cure ensures a uniform degree of monomer conversion throughout the material.

Several studies have been published since the introduction of the dual-cure cements, showing the incapability of the chemically cured cements to compensate for absence of visible light activation even after 24 hours or longer.[25–29] The chemical component of cure in dual-cure resin cements was always found to be lower than the light-cured component, and no evidence was found for a substantial chemically induced polymerization of dual-cured resins after light exposure is completed.[28] A dual-cured resin composite cement that has not been light cured will show incomplete conversion and a porous structure, attributed to incomplete polymerization, which has a negative effect on marginal adaptation.[30] This means that dual-cure cements have the same limitations as do light-activated systems, which are totally dependent on exposure time and light intensity. Ceramic and tooth substance, especially dark and opaque colors and the yellow dentin, attenuate light depending on their thickness and shade. In addition, the inevitable increased distance from the cement results in less complete polymerization.

Clinical Evaluations

It has been established that success with ceramic inlays and onlays can only be achieved when the restorations are permanently bonded to the teeth.[31,32] Attempts at luting ceramic inlays to the tooth with zinc phosphate cement produced high failure rates.[33,34] Bonding of ceramic inlays and onlays to tooth tissues increases resistance to fracture when the ceramic has been etched with hydrofluoric acid or ammonium bifluoride and silane treated.[35] The silane treatment is thought to contribute to covalent bond formation between the ceramic surface and the composite, and it also improves wetting of the ceramic surface by the composite cement. The increased surface roughness of both enamel and ceramic surfaces promotes mechanical interlocking of the composite luting agent to these surfaces.

Light-Cured Resin Composites

A low light intensity of the curing unit led to impaired polymerization of the cured resin cement and adversely affected the resin's physical properties.[36] Also, an increased leakage of unpolymerized resin components can be expected. Inade-

quate depth of cure may reduce the longevity of visible light–activated restorations.[37,38] Isidor and Bröndum[34] reported the durability of fired-ceramic inlays luted with a light-cured resin composite cement followed for 20 to 57 months. An 80% failure rate was observed, and the authors concluded that these cements were not acceptable in clinical practice.[34]

Glass-Ionomer Cements

The use of conventional glass-ionomer luting cements with ceramic inlays was proposed in the early 1990s, especially in deeper cavities with cervical margins in dentin and in patients with high caries activity. An improved chemical bonding of the cement to the tooth should result in improved retention, while a continuous fluoride leakage could give a cariostatic effect. However, in a clinical follow-up, a high frequency of fractured and lost inlays was found for ceramic inlays luted with glass ionomer.[39] In a 6-year split-mouth study of fired feldspathic ceramic inlays (Mirage, Chameleon Dental Products, Kansas City, KS) luted with a conventional glass-ionomer cement and a dual-cure resin composite cement, the glass-ionomer cement–luted inlays showed a significantly higher failure rate.[40] These failures occurred after just 1 year, and the frequency of failed restorations continued to increase during the evaluation (Table 9-1). The glass-ionomer group after 6 years showed a failure rate of 26.3% and the resin group 12.1% (Figs 9-1 and 9-2).[40] After loading, adhesive failures occurred mostly between the fired-ceramic inlay and the glass-ionomer cement (Fig 9-3). The mode of failure showed that the

Table 9-1 Cumulative failure frequencies (%) of fired-ceramic inlays and onlays luted with dual-cured resin composite cement and conventional glass-ionomer cement[40]

Time	Resin composite–luted inlays		Glass-ionomer cement–luted inlays	
	No.	Failures (%)	No.	Failures (%)
Baseline	59	0	59	1.7
6 months	59	1.7	59	3.3
1 year	59	1.7	59	10.2
2 years	59	1.7	59	15.3
3 years	59	3.4	59	15.3
4 years	56	5.4	55	20.0
5 years	56	7.1	55	23.6
6 years	58	12.1	57	26.3

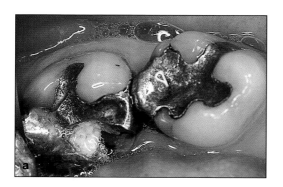

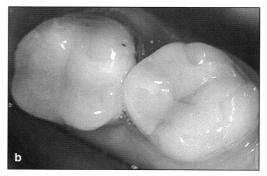

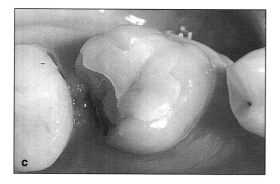

Fig 9-1a Amalgam restorations on teeth 46 and 47 to be replaced by ceramic coverages.

Fig 9-1b Fired-ceramic coverages (Mirage) on teeth 46 and 47 after 1 year. Tooth 46 was luted with a dual-cured resin composite cement, and tooth 47 was luted with a conventional glass-ionomer cement.

Fig 9-1c Partial fracture of the ceramic on tooth 46 after 5 years.

adhesion of the glass-ionomer cement to the etched porcelain was inferior to the micromechanical bonding of the resin composite luting agents.

Two other studies used conventional glass-ionomer cement for luting ceramic inlays. Stenberg and Matsson[41] studied 25 Dicor inlays of limited dimensions dur-

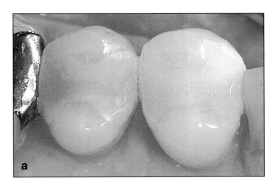
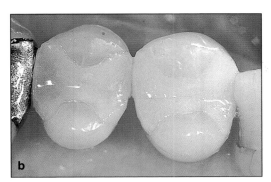

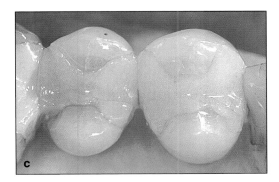

Fig 9-2a Fired-ceramic inlays (Mirage) after luting. The inlay on tooth 14 was luted with glass-ionomer cement, and that on tooth 15 was luted with a dual-cured resin composite.

Fig 9-2b Fired-ceramic inlays after 5 years.

Fig 9-2c Fired-ceramic inlays after 11 years.

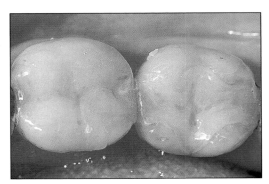
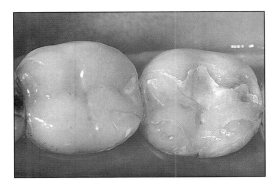

Fig 9-3a The fired-ceramic inlay on tooth 36 was luted with a conventional glass-ionomer cement, and the inlay on tooth 37 was luted with resin composite cement.

Fig 9-3b Partial fracture of the inlay on tooth 36 after 4 years. Adhesive fracture occurred between the ceramic and the glass-ionomer cement.

ing 2 years and reported an 8% failure rate despite the fact that patients with parafunctional habits were excluded. Their preliminary 5-year results showed a failure rate of 23% (Stenberg R, personal communication, 1999. Zuellig and Bryant[30] investigated 35 Cerec inlays (Siemens, Bensheim, Germany) luted with three

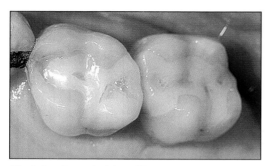

Fig 9-4a Ceramic inlays (Empress) on teeth 26 and 27 after luting. Tooth 26 was luted with a RMGIC, and tooth 27 was luted with a chemically cured resin composite cement.

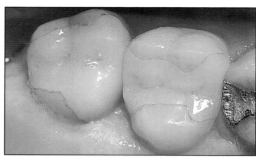

Fig 9-4b Ceramic inlays (Empress) on teeth 16 and 17 after 5 years. Tooth 16 was luted with a chemically cured resin composite and tooth 17 with a RMGIC.

resin composite cements and one glass-ionomer cement. After 3 years, one inlay fractured, and the authors found no differences between the cements. The number of involved inlays was unfortunately low, but it indicates that glass-ionomer cement can function better in ceramics with higher strength.

Resin-Modified Glass-Ionomer Cements

Resin-modified glass ionomer cements show improved mechanical properties compared to conventional glass-ionomer cement. Thoneman et al[42] showed in vitro good marginal integrity of ceramic inlays bonded to dentin with certain RMGICs. They concluded that RMGICs may be an alternative to dentin-bonding agents. Anecdotal reports linked the cement to postcementation fractures, but no clinical controlled study has confirmed this relationship.[16]

A recent study evaluated and compared, intraindividually, IPS Empress ceramic inlays luted with an RMGIC (Fuji Plus, GC, Tokyo, Japan) and a chemically cured resin composite (Panavia 21). Seventy-nine ceramic inlays were placed in Class II cavities in 29 patients.[43] In each patient, half of the inlays were luted with Fuji Plus and the other half with Panavia. The inlays were evaluated clinically, according to modified US Public Health Service criteria,[44] at baseline, after 6 months, and yearly for 5 years. Two small partial fractures were observed at 3 years (one cemented with Panavia, one with Fuji Plus). One inlay (cemented with Panavia) showed recurrent root caries at 4 years. At 5 years, 71 inlays were evaluated. Overall an annual failure rate of 0.2% was observed (Fig 9-4).[43]

It can be concluded that luting with the two chemical-cured luting agents showed a good durability. The RMGIC showed an improved adhesion to etched pressed-ceramic inlays compared to the earlier described luting of fired-ceramic inlays with conventional glass-ionomer cement (Fig 9-5).[40]

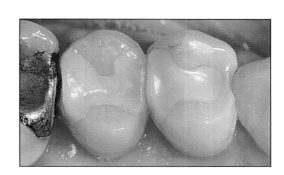

Fig 9-5 Five-year-old Cerec inlays on teeth 14 and 15 luted with chemically cured and dual-cured resin composite cement.

Table 9-2 Clinical evaluations of Class II fired-ceramic inlays luted with dual-cured resin composite cement

Investigator	Year	Evaluation period (y)	No. of inlays	Annual failure rate (%)
van Dijken et al[40]	1998	6	58	2.0
Kanzler and Roulet[45]	1996	6	280	2.5
Molin and Karlsson[46]	1998	5	20	0
Friedl et al[47]	1996	4	96	0
Isodor and Bröndum[34]	1995	3.5	25	2.6
Molin and Karlsson[48]	1996	3	145	4.8
Qualtrough and Wilson[49]	1996	3	–	5.3
Haas et al[50]	1992	2	180	4.4
Christensen et al[51]	1991	2	–	6.0
Jensen et al[52]	1988	2	9	1.2

Dual-Cured Resin Composites

Dual-cured resin composites became popular with the assumption that an optimal conversion could be obtained in deeper parts of the cavity. Studies of fired-ceramic inlays luted with dual-cured resin composite luting agents showed a large variation in failure rates (Table 9-2). The main reasons for failure were total or

Table 9-3 Clinical evaluations of Class II pressed-ceramic inlays luted with dual-cured resin composite cements

Investigator	Year	Evaluation period (y)	No. of inlays	Annual failure rate (%)
Frankenberger et al[55]	1999	6	59	1.2
van Dijken et al[5]	2001	5	78	0.2
Krämer et al[56]	1999	4	96	1.8
Molin and Karlsson[46]	1998	5	20	4.0
Studer et al[57]	1998	6	163	1.2
Fradeani et al[58]	1997	3	125	1.6
Tidehag and Gunne[59]	1995	2	62	0.9
Reinelt et al[60]	1995	2	96	1.6

partial fracture of the inlays resulting from insufficient retention of the cement to the ceramic material. No or very low secondary caries frequencies were observed. The large variations in failure rates may be the result of many factors, such as type of ceramic material, technique sensitivity, influence of operator, and operative procedure, including preparation depth and form, mode of luting, and type of luting agent. In some studies, patients with signs of clenching, bruxism, poor oral hygiene, or high caries risk were excluded; the patients included do not reflect the patient population of general dentists.[34,47]

High failure rates were reported for Dicor inlays luted with resin composite: 6% after 2 years,[41] 10% after 4 to 82 months, and 13% after 4 years.[41,51,53,54] Glass ionomer–luted inlays showed a failure rate of 8% after 2 years and 23% after 5 years.[41]

The injection-molded, leucite-reinforced ceramic material Empress has been reported to undergo less shrinkage, show less porosity, and be less brittle than conventional feldspathic ceramics. Clinical evaluations of Empress inlays luted with dual-cured resin composites showed an increased durability compared to fired-ceramic inlays (Table 9-3).

Chemically Cured Materials

To ensure an optimal conversion in the entire cement layer, chemical luting agents have been suggested. Disadvantages of these materials are the relatively short working time, which, however, should be sufficient when placing single reconstructions. Mixing causes air bubbles to be incorporated in the paste-paste resin and has been named a disadvantage. A reduction of polymerization stress due to a slower hardening time can optimize the marginal adaptation and decrease risk for postoperative sensitivity.[61–65]

Doubts about the setting of the dual-cured resin composite luting agents led to clinical studies in our research group.

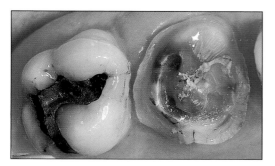

Fig 9-6a Nonretentive preparation for an enamel-dentin–bonded ceramic complete coverage on tooth 16.

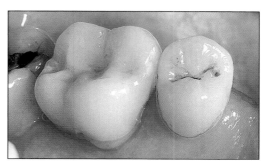

Fig 9-6b Enamel-dentin–bonded ceramic crown (Empress), luted with a chemically cured resin composite, after 6 years.

In one study, each of 27 patients received two Cerec inlays, one luted with a chemically cured composite material (Cavex Clearfil F2, Haarlem, The Netherlands) and the other with a dual-cured resin composite (Vita Cerec Duo cement, Coltène, Altstätten, Switzerland). At 5 years a higher fracture rate was found in the dual-cured resin group, but the differences were not significant (see Fig 9-5).[66] At 10 years, the survival rate was 77% for the dual cured resin composite–luted inlays and 100% for the chemically cured resin composite–luted inlays. [67]

In a recent study of extensive dentin-enamel–bonded posterior partial and complete-coverage ceramic restorations, the effect of luting with a dual-cured and a self-cured luting agent was studied.[5] In 110 patients, 182 complete-coverage ceramic restorations (IPS Empress) were placed between November 1992 and December 1996. Adhesive bonding to dentin and enamel was performed with three bonding systems. In 58 restorations the classic Syntac (Ivoclar Vivadent) was used in combination with the dual-cured resin composite Variolink (Ivoclar Vivadent). In the other restorations luted with the chemically-cured resin composite Bisfil 2B (Bisco, Chicago, IL), 25 were bonded with the classic Gluma (Bayer, Dormhagen, Germany), 57 with Allbond 2 (Bisco), and 42 with Syntac (Fig 9-6). Of the 182 ceramic restorations, 13 (7.1%) were evaluated as unacceptable after a mean observation of 4.9 years (range 4.3 to 7.5 years). The reasons for failure were fracture (5), lost restorations (4), secondary caries (3), and endodontic treatment (1). No significant differences in failure rate were seen between the two luting agents nor between the three dentin-bonding agents.[5]

Ditching

It has been stated[30] that degradation of a luting cement by wear should be the weak link in ceramic and resin composite inlays and can jeopardize the durability of the restoration. Ditching, the result of the wear of the luting agent in the joint between the tooth and the inlay, has been associated with leakage at the interface, which could result in marginal discoloration and secondary caries. In one study, ditching was already detectable with indirect evaluation techniques at the 8-month recall appointments.[22]

The wear of the cement can be quickened as a result of incomplete curing, premature removal of the excess cement, and/or abrasion of an oxygen-inhibited surface layer with relatively lower abrasion resistance. Cement wear has been reported in almost all clinical evaluations of ceramic inlays. Several studies have investigated the influence of the type of luting agent or the widths of the margins on the degree of wear. In some studies, microfilled resin composites have shown a superior clinical wear resistance in short time evaluations compared to hybrid resin composites, while other studies found no difference.[22,40] However, for marginal leakage to occur, ditching alone is not enough; marginal crack or gap formation must also be present. Ditching was not found to be a clinical problem in any of the published clinical follow-up studies.[5,20,22,40,43,45,55,56,58,66] Clinical evaluation and scanning electron microscopy results show that the loss of luting material seems to occur mostly during the first years after placement and then levels off and probably remains stable when the ditching reaches a certain depth.[22,40,50] It has been suggested that toothbrush bristles are unable to reach and abrade the cement in the bottom of a deep gap, which would slow down or almost arrest the ditching process successively. Only a slight proximal marginal wear was reported in several long-term studies, indicating ditching to be an occlusal problem probably caused by wear via food bolus.[22,40,55,58] Marginal wear does not result in significant clinical risk or an increased number of failed inlays.

Secondary Caries

Secondary caries has been reported to be the main reason for failure of most restorative procedures. For ceramic inlays the frequency of secondary caries is far lower. Of a review of 2- to 3-year evaluations, 15 of 20 studies did not show secondary caries contiguous to the inlays.[40] In 5 other studies, frequencies of between 0.5% and 4.7% were seen. In the 4- to 5-year evaluations, 4 studies did not report secondary caries, while 1 study reported 5.1%. In a 6-year study, in which 46% of the involved patients had a high caries risk, a 2.6% secondary caries frequency was observed.[40] The majority of 182 extensive dentin-enamel–bonded complete-coverage ceramic restorations in a 5-year follow-up had their cervical margins located in dentin. Only a few of these showed secondary caries or marginal discoloration, which confirms the sealing ability of dentin-bonded ceramic restorations. It can be suggested from the reported inlay studies that inlays are a good treatment option for caries-active patients if prophylactic measures are followed. This has also been reported in long-term evaluations of resin composite inlays.

Conclusions

Phosphate cements, light-cured resin composites, and conventional glass-ionomer cements showed unacceptable, high clinical failure rates and are not suitable for luting dental ceramic inlays. Dual-cured and chemically cured resin composites and a RMGIC showed better durability. Inlays of pressed ceramics and CAD/CAM produced ceramics showed better longevity than did fired ceramics. Concerning the high annual failure rate of fired-ceramic inlays and the favorable performance of resin composite in Class II cavities, the clinical indication of Class II inlays is not advisable.

References

1. Hench LL. Bioceramics. From concept to clinic. J Am Ceram Soc 1991;74:1487–1510.

2. Peters MCRB, de Vree JHP, Brekelmans WAM. Distributed crack analysis of ceramic inlays. J Dent Res 1993;72:1537–1542.

3. Van Dijken JWV. All-ceramic restoratives: Classification and clinical evaluations. Compend Contin Educ Dent 1999;20:1115–1134.

4. Nakabayashi N, Nakamuru M, Yasuda N. Hybrid layer as a dentin-bonding mechanism. J Esthet Dent 1991;3:133–138.

5. Van Dijken JWV, Hasselrot L, Örmin A, Olofsson A-L. Durability of extensive dentin-enamel–bonded ceramic coverages (IPS Empress). A 5-year follow-up. Eur J Oral Sci 2001;109:1–8.

6. Rosenblom MA, Schulman A. A review of all-ceramic restorations. J Am Dent Assoc 1997; 128:297–307.

7. Anusavice KJ, Lee RB. Effect of firing temperature and water exposure on crack propagation in unglazed porcelain. J Dent Res 1989;68: 1075–1081.

8. Denry IL. Recent advances in ceramics for dentistry. Crit Rev Oral Biol Med 1996;7:134–143.

9. Anusavice KJ. Recent developments in restorative dental ceramics. J Am Dent Assoc 1993; 124:72–84.

10. Dong JK, Lüthy H, Wohlwend A, Schärer P. Heat-pressed ceramics: Technology and strength. Int J Prosthodont 1992;5:9–16.

11. Chan KC, Svare CV, Harton DJ. The effect of varnish on dentinal bonding strength of five dental cements. J Prosthet Dent 1976;35: 403–406.

12. Schwartz NL, Whitsett LD, Berry TG, Stewart JL. Unserviceable crowns and fixed partial dentures: Life-span and causes for loss of serviceability. J Am Dent Assoc 1970;81:1395–1401.

13. Johnson GH, Powell LV, Derouen DA. Evaluation and control of post-cementation pulpal sensitivity: Zinc phosphate cement and glass-ionomer luting cements. J Am Dent Assoc 1993;112:654–657.

14. Brackett WW, Metz JE. Performance of a glass-ionomer luting cement in a general practice. J Prosthet Dent 1992;67:59–61.

15. Van Dijken JWV. Durability of new restorative materials in Class III cavities. J Adhes Dent 2001;3:65–70.

16. Miller MB. Resin-ionomer luting agents. Reality Now 1995;(July).

17. Leevailoj C, Platt JA, Cochran A, Moore BK. In vitro study of fracture incidence and compressive fracture load of all-ceramic crowns cemented with resin-modified glass ionomer and other luting agents. J Prosthet Dent 1998;80:699–707.

18. Van Dijken J, Lundin S-Å, Paulander J. Dentala Kompositer. Jönköping, Sweden: LIC förlag AB, 1992.

19. Davidson CL, van Zeghbroeck, Feilzer AJ. Destructive stresses in adhesive luting cements. J Dent Res 1991;70:880–882.

20. Van Dijken JWV, Hörstedt P. Marginal breakdown of 5-year-old direct composite inlays. J Dent 1996;24:389–394.

21. Shortall AC, Fayyad MA, Williams JD. Marginal seal of injection-molded crowns cemented with three different adhesive systems. J Prosthet Dent 1989;61:24–27.

22. Pallesen U, van Dijken JWV. An 8-year evaluation of sintered ceramic and glass ceramic inlays processed by the Cerec CAD/CAM system. Eur J Oral Sci 2000;108:239–246.

23. White SN. Adhesive cements and cementation. J Calif Dent Assoc 1993;21:30–37.

24. Watts DC, Cash AJ. Analysis of optical transmission by 400–500 μm visible light into aesthetic dental biomaterials. J Dent 1994;22: 112–117.

25. Blackman R, Barghi N, Duke E. Influence of ceramic thickness on the polymerization of light-cured resin cements. J Prosthet Dent 1990;63: 295–300.

26. Breeding LC, Dixon DL, Caughman WF. The curing potential of light-activated composite resin luting agents. J Prosthet Dent 1991;65: 512–518.

27. Hasagawa EA, Boyer DB, Chan DC. Hardening of dual-cured cements under composite resin inlays. J Prosthet Dent 1991;66:187–192.

28. Rueggeberg FA, Caughman WF. The influence of light exposure on polymerization of dual-cure resin cements. Oper Dent 1993;18:48–55.

29. Uctasli S, Hasanreisoglu U, Wilson HJ. The attenuation of radiation by porcelain and its effect on polymerization of resin cements. J Oral Rehab 1994;21:565–575.

30. Zuellig R, Bryant RW. Three-year clinical evaluation of luting agents for Cerec restorations [abstract 1042]. J Dent Res 1996;75:148.

31. Feilzer AJ, De Gee AJ, Davidson CL. Increased wall-to-wall curing contraction in thin bonded resin layers. J Dent Res 1989;68:48–50.

32. Feilzer AJ, De Gee AJ, Davidson CL. Setting stress in composite resin in relation to configuration of the restoratives. J Dent Res 1987;66:1636–1639.

33. Banks RG. Conservative posterior ceramic restorations: A literature review. J Prosthet Dent 1990;63:619–626.

34. Isidor F, Bröndum K. A clinical evaluation of porcelain inlays. J Prosthet Dent 1995;74:140–144.

35. Dietschi D, Maeder M, Meyer J-M, Holz J. In vitro resistance to fracture of porcelain inlays bonded to tooth. Quintessence Int 1990;21:823–831.

36. Ferracane JL, Greener EH. The effect of resin formulation on the degree of conversion and mechanical properties of dental restorative resins. J Biomed Mater Res 1986;20:121–131.

37. Feilzer AJ, Dooren LH, De Gee AJ, Davidson CL. Influence of light intensity on polymerization shrinkage and integrity of restoration-cavity interface. Eur J Oral Sci 1995;103:322–326.

38. Shortall AC, Wilson HJ, Harrington E. Depth of cure of radiation-activated composite restoratives. Influence of shade and opacity. J Oral Rehabil 1995;22:337–342.

39. Höglund-Åberg C, van Dijken JWV, Olofsson AL. Three-year comparison of fired ceramic inlays cemented with composite resin or glass-ionomer cement. Acta Odontol Scand 1994;52:140–149.

40. Van Dijken JWV, Höglund-Åberg C, Olofsson AL. Fired ceramic inlays. A 6-year follow-up. J Dent 1998;26:219–225.

41. Stenberg R, Matsson L. Clinical evaluation of glass-ceramic inlays (Dicor). Acta Odontol Scand 1993;51:91–97.

42. Thoneman B, Federlin M, Schmalz G, Hiller K-A. Resin-modified glass ionomers for luting posterior ceramic restorations. Dent Mater 1995;11:161–168.

43. Van Dijken JWV. Resin-modified glass-ionomer cement and self-cured resin composite luted ceramic inlays. A 5-year clinical evaluation. Dent Mater 2003;19:670–674.

44. Van Dijken JWV. A clinical evaluation of anterior conventional, microfiller and hybrid composite resin fillings. Acta Odontol Scand 1986;44:357–367.

45. Kanzler R, Roulet J-F. Margin quality and longevity in vivo of sintered ceramic inlays luted with adhesive techniques. In: Mörmann WH (ed) CAD/CIM in Aesthetic Dentistry. Chicago: Quintessence, 1996:537–552.

46. Molin M, Karlsson S. A 5-year clinical evaluation of three ceramic inlay systems [abstract 2252]. J Dent Res 1998;77:913.

47. Friedl KH, Schmalz G, Hiller KA, Saller A. In vivo evaluation of a feldspathic ceramic system: 2-year results. J Dent 1996;24:25–31.

48. Molin M, Karlsson S. A 3-year follow-up study of a ceramic Optec inlay system. Acta Odontol Scand 1996;51:145–149.

49. Qualtrough AJE, Wilson NHF. A 3-year clinical evaluation of a porcelain inlay system. J Dent 1996;24:317–323.

50. Haas M, Arnetzl G, Wegscheider WA, König K, Bratschka RO. Clinical and material behavior of composite, ceramic, and gold inlays [in German]. Dtsch Zahnartzl Z 1992;47:18–22.

51. Christensen R, Christensen G, Vogl S, Bangerter V. 2-year clinical comparison of 6 inlay systems [abstract 2360]. J Dent Res 1991;70:561.

52. Jensen ME. A 2-year clinical study of posterior etched-porcelain resin-bonded restorations. Am J Dent 1988;1:27–33.

53. Noack MJ, Roulet JF. Survival rates and mode of failure of Dicor inlays after 4 years [abstract 759]. J Dent Res 1994;73:196.

54. Roulet JF. The longevity of glass-ceramic inlays [abstract 36]. J Dent Res 1995;74:405.

55. Frankenberger R, Petschelt A, Krämer N. Leucite-reinforced glass-ceramic inlays and onlays after 6 years: Clinical behavior. Oper Dent 2000;25:459–465.

56. Krämer N, Frankenberger R, Pelka M, Petschelt A. IPS Empress inlays and onlays after 4 years—A clinical study. J Dent 1999;27:325–331.

57. Studer S, Lehner C, Schärer P. Seven-year results of leucite-reinforced glass-ceramic inlays and onlays [abstract 1375]. J Dent Res 1998; 77:803.

58. Fradeani M, Aquilano A, Bassein L. Longitudinal study of pressed glass-ceramic inlays for four and a half years. J Prosthet Dent 1997;78:346–353.

59. Tidehag P, Gunne J. A 2-year clinical follow-up study of IPS Empress ceramic inlays. Int J Prosthodont 1995:456–460.

60. Reinelt C, Krämer N, Pelka M, Petschelt A. In vivo performance of IPS Empress inlays and onlays after 2 years [abstract 1211]. J Dent Res 1995;74:552.

61. Davidson CL, De Gee AJ. Relaxation of polymerization contraction stresses by flow in dental composites. J Dent Res 1984;63:146–148.

62. Feilzer AJ, De Gee AJ, Davidson CL. Quantative determination of stress reduction by flow in composite restorations. Dent Mater 1990;6: 167–171.

63. Goodis HE, White JM, Gamm B, Watanabe L. Pulp chamber temperature changes with visible-light–cured composites in vitro. Dent Mater 1990;6:99–102.

64. Goodis HE, White JM, Marshall SJ, Koshrovi P, Watanabe LG, Marshall GW Jr. The effect of glass-ionomer liners in lowering pulp temperatures during composite placement in vitro. Dent Mater 1993;9:146–150.

65. Itoh K, Yanagawa T, Wakumoto S. Effect of composition and curing type of composite on adaptation to dentin cavity walls. Dent Mater J 1986;5:260–266.

66. Sjögren G, Molin M, van Dijken JWV. A 5-year clinical evaluation of ceramic inlays (Cerec) cemented with a dual-cured or a chemically cured luting agent. Acta Odontol Scand 1998;56: 263–267.

67. Sjögren G, Molin M, van Dijken JWV. A 10-year prospective evaluation of CAD/CAM-manufactured (Cerec) ceramic inlays cemented with a chemically cured or dual-cured resin composite. Int J Prosthodont 2004;17:241–246.

Chapter 10

An Overview of the Clinical Use of Resin-to-Metal Bonding

Richard van Noort

Abstract

Rapid expansion in the materials and procedures available for resin-to-metal bonding has broadened its application in dentistry. In this chapter various aspects of the clinical application of this new technology are explored in the context of their use in dental surgery. The different requirements for base metal alloy and precious metal alloy bonding are considered. Issues related to the selection of luting resin for resin-bonded prostheses are addressed, and the different methods of precious metal bonding are examined. A number of recommendations are made as to the best materials and procedures to use under which circumstances and are intended to provoke a debate.

The ability to bond resins to metals is of growing clinical interest, as indicated by the ever-expanding range of dental applications. These include:

- Resin instead of ceramic veneers on metal substructures
- Resin-bonded orthodontic brackets
- Bonding of minimal-preparation resin-retained prostheses
- Resin-bonded endodontic metal posts
- Resin bonding of conventional fixed partial dentures where there is compromised retention
- Intraoral repair of ceramic fractures on metal-ceramic restorations
- Amalgam bonding

All of these clinical applications of resin-to-metal bonding represent a considerable challenge, both scientifically and practically. As in all areas of dentistry, especially the area of dental materials, it should come as no surprise that many new surface treatments and new resin adhesives have become available in recent years.

To improve the bond between the metal and the resin, a wide variety of approaches have been explored. Initially these involved the use of macroscopic retentive features such as beads, but gradually, adhesive procedures involving micromechanical and/or chemical bonding were developed. The latter can be accomplished with a resin adhesive that has functional groups that can bond directly to the metal. Another approach is the use of adhesion promoters such as silica coating, tin plating, and tribochemical coatings. Metal primers have been developed to improve the bond between the metal and conventional bisphenol glycidyl methacrylate (bis-GMA)– or urethane dimethacrylate (UDMA)–based resins. An added complication is that the efficacy of many of these procedures depends on whether the clinician is seeking to bond to a base metal alloy or a precious metal alloy. In fact, it is convenient to consider the issue of resin-to-metal bonding as falling into these two fundamental areas. While there has been a parallel development of resin-to-metal bonding systems and materials for both laboratory and clinical use, this chapter will focus on the clinical rather than the laboratory use of resin-to-metal bonding.

Base Metal Alloy Bonding

Macromechanical Bonding

Since the 1940s, dental laboratories have used resin veneers on removable and fixed partial dentures. At that time the resin was polymethyl methacrylate, which was attached to the metal framework by macromechanical retention. Problems arose because the resin would not adapt well to the metal because of the extensive polymerization shrinkage of the methyl methacrylate, resulting in the formation of microgaps, discoloration, and eventually loosening and fracture.[1,2] With the arrival of metal-ceramic restorations in the 1960s many of these problems were in effect overcome and ceramic veneers became the preferred choice for fixed partial dentures, while acrylic resin continued to be used for removable partial dentures. It was not until the 1980s that there was a resurgence of interest in using resins as veneers on metal substructures as an alternative to ceramics. Visible light–activated resin composite veneers on metal restorations have become popular because of easy handling, a hardness not dissimilar to that of enamel, and excellent esthetics of veneering composite.[3] This coincided with other improvements in resin composites, which had become much stronger and more wear resistant. However, effective bonding of these resins to metal was still a serious problem.[4]

In the meantime, clinically similar problems were experienced with the resin bonding of metal structures directly to the teeth. In 1973, Rochette[5] first reported the use of metal structures that were bonded by resins to acid-etched enamel. He used thin, perforated metal castings, bonded with cold-cure acrylic resins, to splint mobile mandibular incisors that were affected by advanced bone loss. Following the successful retention of these devices, he then had the idea of adding a pontic to the splint where a missing tooth needed to be replaced. This provided a means of replac-

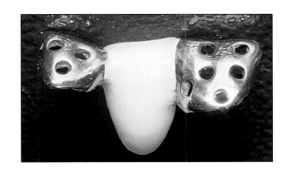

Fig 10-1 Rochette bridge. (Courtesy of Dr S. Northeast.)

ing a missing tooth that involved minimal tooth preparation (Fig 10-1). One weakness of the so-called Rochette bridge design was the use of small perforations for retention. This design exposed the resin to wear and also meant that the resin was attached to a relatively small area of the metal retainer.[6] Alternative macroretentive features, such as beads, wires, or loops in the metal design, originally explored in the dental laboratory for the metal frameworks with acrylic veneers, did not resolve the problem. Although less resin was exposed and thus wear would not be such a problem, the bulky framework required to accommodate these macroretentive features remained a problem.[7] Thus an improved method of bonding resin to the metal was needed.

Micromechanical Bonding

The problem of having to rely on macroretentive features was overcome to some degree in the early 1980s when a new method of treating nickel-chromium (Ni-Cr) alloys was developed.[8,9] With this method, the entire fitting surface of the retainer is rendered micromechanically retentive by either electrolytic or acid-gel etching. However, this technique is only applicable to certain alloys, such as Ni-Cr or cobalt-chromium (Co-Cr), which have a heterogeneous microstructure (Fig 10-2). The light and dark regions represent areas with a different composition (phase), and the etching process preferentially removes one of these phases, which results in a pitted and grooved surface appearance (Fig 10-3). This technique provides a highly retentive surface such that the luting resin adheres strongly to the metal surface as a result of the high degree of micromechanical interlocking introduced. It bonds the entire area of the retainer to the etched enamel and protects the underlying resin. Retainer design can be made by waxing directly onto investment models, resulting in an accurate fit. This was the basis of the so-called Maryland bridge, although with the advent of other methods of achieving a resin-to-metal bond, other terms such as *resin-bonded prostheses* or *minimal preparation prostheses* are now commonly used.

The luting resins used with these prostheses are essentially very similar to composite resin restorative materials, consisting of a bis-GMA or UDMA resin and glass filler. Since access of light to the

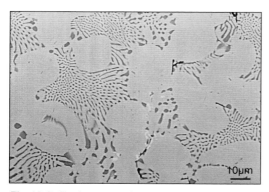

Fig 10-2 Back-scattered scanning electron microscope image (SEM) of the polished surface of a Ni-Cr alloy, showing the compositional variation.

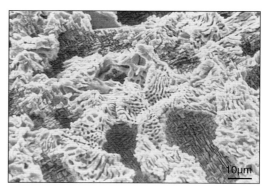

Fig 10-3 SEM of the etched surface of a Ni-Cr alloy.

resin is restricted by the metal retainers, these resins differ from the restorative composites in that they are invariably two-paste chemically cured or dual-cure systems. The filler particle size is less than 20 μm, and the filler loading tends to be slightly lower to ensure a low film thickness. An optical opacifier such as titanium oxide may be added to prevent metal show-through.

Nevertheless, a number of drawbacks soon became apparent[10]:

- Electroetching requires a high degree of skill and specialized equipment.
- Although a gel-etching process gradually replaced the electroetching process, these gels are high concentration solutions of strong acids, which are highly toxic and need to be handled with great care.
- Beryllium is present in some Ni-Cr alloys to improve castability and to provide a superior etch pattern. However, beryllium is highly toxic in its free state and may be released during grinding

and polishing of the castings. Therefore, dental laboratories prefer to use beryllium-free alloys, which unfortunately do not etch as well.
- It is not possible to judge with the naked eye if the appropriate etch pattern has been achieved, even under magnification with an optical microscope.
- The technique is limited to certain alloys and is not applicable to intraoral repair.

Chemically Adhesive Resins

To comply with the wishes of dental laboratories not wanting to use beryllium-containing Ni-Cr alloys and with a desire to avoid the etching process, some other means of bonding to the alloy had to be found. The bis-GMA– and UDMA-type resins do not adhere well to untreated metal surfaces, relying primarily on micromechanical adhesion. Airborne-particle abrasion of base metal alloys with 50-μm alumina grit produces some surface

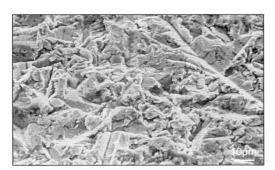

Fig 10-4 SEM of the airborne particle–abraded surface of a Ni-Cr alloy.

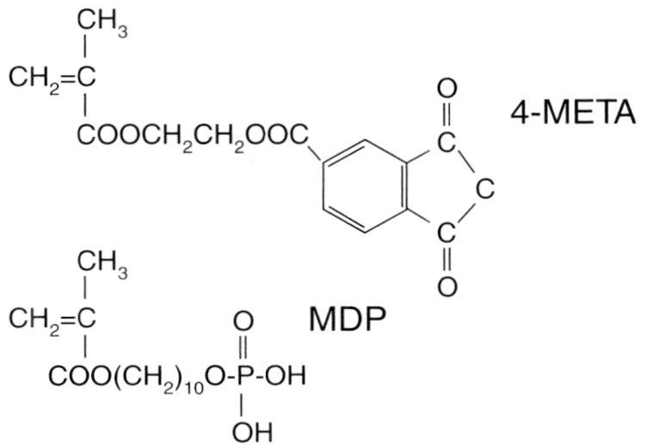

Fig 10-5 Structure of 4-META and MDP resins.

roughening for micromechanical adhesion (Fig 10-4). However, the surface does not have the reentrant features associated with the etched surface and provides inadequate micromechanical adhesion. Hence, the bis-GMA– or UDMA-based resin composite cannot be used directly on airborne particle–abraded Ni-Cr alloy surfaces, as the bond is not sufficiently strong for these resins.[11]

To improve the adhesive bond of resins to the metal surface, a variety of luting resins have been developed in which the resin component has been modified to bond chemically to suitably prepared metal surfaces by the incorporation of organic esters.[1,12] These luting resins are generally referred to as *chemically adhesive luting resins* to differentiate them from the bis-GMA–type resins. In one such system, the active constituent is the carboxylic monomer 4-methacryloxyethyl trimellitate anhydride (4-META), commercially available as C&B Superbond (Sun Medical, Shiga, Japan). Another luting resin has been modified

to incorporate a phosphate monomer (methacryloxyethyl-phenyl phosphate, MDP). An example of this type of resin is Panavia 21 (Kuraray, Osaka, Japan). Resin bonding is facilitated by the high affinity of resins containing carboxylic acid or phosphoric acid derivatives for the metal oxide on the base metal alloy (Fig 10-5). These resins have been shown to provide a durable bond to the airborne particle–abraded metal surface of Ni-Cr and Co-Cr alloys.[13–16] Therefore, there is no need for etching and thus no need for special laboratory equipment or the use of dangerous chemical reagents. With the advent of these resins, it is now possible to form a strong chemically adhesive bond between an airborne particle–abraded base metal alloy and acid-etched enamel.

There is still the issue of which of the two types of adhesive luting resin is the most effective. This will depend to a large extent on the type of application being considered, but because these resins are used extensively for the cementation of

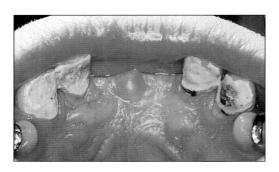

Fig 10-6 Debonded resin-bonded prosthesis. (Courtesy of Dr S. Northeast.)

resin-bonded prostheses, this is an application worth exploring further. The adhesive resins are popular precisely because of their adhesive qualities. Nevertheless, debonding of resin-bonded prostheses is a common mode of failure.[17] The general view is, quite reasonably, that the higher the bond strength of the resin to the metal, the less likely it will be that the resin-bonded prosthesis will debond. In a tensile bond strength test carried out by Degrange and Attal,[18] an MDP-based adhesive showed a bond strength nearly three times greater than that of a 4-META–based resin, 71 and 28 MPa respectively, and well above that of the resin-bond to enamel. However, does this mean that the MDP-based luting resin will perform better? With retainers having a surface area of approximately 10 mm², the tensile force required to cause a debond would have to be in the region of 300 to 700 N. Such high forces on a resin-bonded prosthesis are very unlikely. So, if they adhere so well to the metal, why do resin-bonded prostheses debond, and why does this debond typically occur at the metal-resin interface rather than at the enamel-resin interface (Fig 10-6)? An interesting observation made by Creugers and Käyser[17] was that prostheses that had debonded were considerably more likely to debond again after re-bonding, suggesting that the problem is more fundamental than what at first glance appears to be merely a lack of adhesion.

In the case of resin-bonded prostheses, the adhesive plays a dual role. That is, it has to bond the metal to the tooth, and it also has to transfer the load applied to the prosthesis across the adhesive into the tooth. Since the prosthesis acts essentially as a beam bonded to the tooth surface, the adhesive layer will need to be able to resist a considerable amount of stress,[19,20] and this suggests that a structural adhesive is required. That is, the adhesive not only has to bond well to the metal and the tooth, but it also has to be sufficiently strong to withstand the stresses within the adhesive layer. For example, glass-ionomer cements produce an excellent bond to enamel and dentin but make poor adhesives because of their lack of strength. In addition, inherent in the design of a resin-bonded prosthesis are highly local-

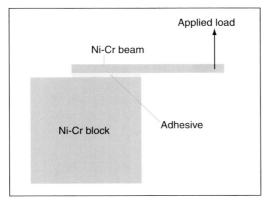

Fig 10-7 Schematic of the tensile peel strength test arrangement.

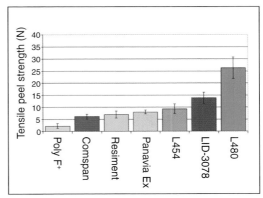

Fig 10-8 Tensile peel strength data for a range of adhesives with increasing fracture toughness, including a dental cement (Poly F+ [Dentsply, Weybridge, UK]), three luting resins (Comspan [Kerr UK, Peterborough, UK], Resiment [Septodont, New Castle, DE], and Panavia Ex [Kuraray]), and three experimental adhesives (L454, LID-3078, L480) provided by Loctite International (Dublin, Ireland).

ized stresses in the region of the connector, such that the adhesive has to be able to not only withstand very high stresses but also resist the propagation of cracks from any internal or surface defects. This means that the adhesive needs to be tough. However, most dental adhesives are brittle due to the nature of the resins used and the incorporation of particulate fillers. This aspect of the behavior of adhesives is frequently overlooked.

The concept of a tensile peel strength as a means of comparing the adhesive capabilities of luting resins was explored in a study by Northeast et al[20] in which a beam was bonded to a simple support structure (Fig 10-7). This study showed that the tensile peel strength was a function of the thickness of the beam, such that the thicker the beam, the less the tensile peel force. With a thicker beam the level of stress within the adhesive layer was reduced. This demonstrates that the stress the adhesive has to withstand is an important contributory factor to the clinical outcome and is governed by the choice of alloy and its design. Northeast et al[20] also showed that the tensile peel force depended on the choice of luting resin. When a series of materials with increasing toughness were tested using the tensile peel strength test, it was found that, irrespective of their ability to bond to the metal, the tensile peel force increases as the fracture toughness of the adhesive is increased (Fig 10-8). Interestingly, Degrange and Attal[18] showed that the 4-META–based luting resin is tougher than many other luting resins. It has also been reported that the 4-META–based resin caused fewer debonds of resin-bonded prostheses than when a more brittle bis-

GMA–based resin was used.[21] This would seem to suggest that, at least for resin-bonded prostheses, a high-toughness adhesive resin would produce superior clinical results compared with a relatively more brittle adhesive resin, assuming both are able to produce an adequate and durable bond to the metal.

Despite these observations the MDP-based adhesive resin tends to be more popular with many dental practitioners because of its superior handling characteristics (paste-paste) compared to the 4-META–based resin (powder-liquid). This merely confirms the old adage that producing the best possible dental material is no good unless dental practitioners like the handling characteristics. Thus the immediate and perfectly achievable challenge would seem to be to produce a very tough adhesive with optimum handling characteristics for use with resin-bonded prostheses. Nevertheless, it would appear that a strong and durable bond to base metal alloys is possible with the chemically adhesive luting resins.

Precious Metal Alloy Bonding

At the same time that adhesive techniques were being developed to improve the bonding to base metal alloys, there was a growing desire among dental practitioners to bond resins to precious metal alloys. Partly this was driven by a desire to undertake intraoral repairs of metal-ceramic restorations, in which the ceramic had separated from the metal substructure, and avoid costly remakes. However, by the 1990s the problem of bonding to dentin had, to a

large extent, been overcome with the introduction of reasonably effective dentin bonding agents. Hence there was also a growing desire to bond precious metal crowns and fixed partial dentures with resin, especially in situations of compromised retention, such as short clinical crowns.

While chemically adhesive luting resins are excellent for bonding to base metal alloys, they have a relatively low affinity for precious metal alloys such as gold and palladium because of the lack of a surface oxide coating. This low chemical reactivity of the surface of precious metal alloys may be overcome by surface modification to make it more amenable to forming a bond with a luting resin or an esthetic restorative resin composite. Three popular options have become available:

- Application of a more reactive coating to the surface by electrodeposition, eg, tin plating
- Alteration of the surface chemistry by silica coating
- Application of a specially formulated metal primer

Tin Plating

The concept of tin plating was introduced to dentistry as far back as 1977 to allow bonding of polyacrylic acid cements to precious metal alloys.[22] A technique for tin plating precious metal alloys chairside has since been developed, and two systems are commercially available (Micro Tin, Danville Engineering, San Ramon, CA; and Kura Ace Mini, J. Morita, Osaka, Japan). The procedure deposits a layer of tin on the precious metal alloy surface; it can be seen by the appear-

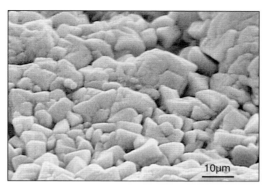

Fig 10-9 Tin-plated surface of a palladium alloy.

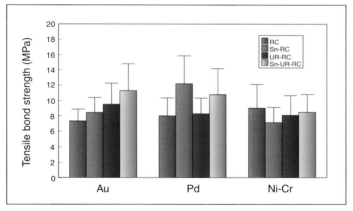

Fig 10-10 Effect of tin plating on the tensile bond strength of gold, palladium, and Ni-Cr alloys. (RC) Resin control; (Sn) tin plated; (UR) unfilled resin.

ance of a gray discoloration. The surface layer produced is irregular in form and provides some degree of micromechanical retention for the resins (Fig 10-9).

Although laboratory data suggest that there is an improvement in the bond strength of bis-GMA– and UDMA-based resins to a tin-plated precious metal alloy,[23,24] this has also been found to be alloy specific.[25,26] Other results[27] suggest that the improvement for resin composites bonded directly to the tin-plated surface is only marginal and better methods of bonding such resins to precious metal alloys are required (Fig 10-10). The results with chemically adhesive resins are possibly more promising since these resins provide a chemical bond to the tin oxide,[28] whereas the more conventional resins rely essentially on a process of micromechanical interlocking.

There are also some possible drawbacks with tin plating. It has been suggested that the application of an excessively thick layer of tin plating can result in a low bond strength because the oxide coating is too thick.[29] Thus, the procedure for tin plating is critical and potentially subject to error. In addition, there may be clinical situations, such as intraoral repairs, in which the alloy is unknown. If the exposed metal is a Ni-Cr alloy, then tin plating provides no benefit and may even be detrimental to obtaining a strong resin bond.

Silica Coating

The use of silane coupling agents to enhance adhesion of dental ceramics to tooth structure via a resin composite is well established. The possibility of silanating cast metals is limited due to a lack of appropriate binding sites on the alloy surface.[30] It is now possible to produce a silica coating on metal surfaces, making them amenable to silane coupling and successful resin bonding. Two techniques are available, one involving a special coating and heat-treatment technique of the alloy and the other involving a tribochemical approach.

Silicoater

The Silicoater system (Kulzer, Friedrichsdorf, Germany) requires the metal surface to be passed through a propane-air flame, in which tetramethoxysilane is decomposed. As a result an intermediary layer of SiO_x is formed—providing Si-OH groups for silane bonding. A silane cou-

pling agent is applied to this silicoated surface, which is able to bond with the resin.[31,32] Since this is a dental laboratory procedure, it will not be considered further here, although it should be said that there is overwhelming evidence that the bond to base metal alloys, including titanium, is significantly improved with this system.[33,34]

Tribochemical coating

In this technique, the alloy surface is airborne-particle abraded at high pressure with a special powder that contains fine alumina and colloidal silica particles. The technique was first introduced in the late 1980s as a laboratory-based system for improving the bond of acrylic resins to metallic frameworks[12,35,36] and is called Rocatec (3M Espe, Seefeld, Germany).

The objective is to form a thin layer of silica on the metal surface, which contains sufficient free hydroxyl (–OH) groups to allow coupling to resin via a silane coupling agent. This technique is known as *tribochemical silica coating*, as it has been shown that particles, impacting the alloy surface at high speed, can cause transfer of a silica layer to the metal. This layer is said to be stable (Fig 10-11). This pretreated surface is then silane treated and is ready for resin bonding. As with the Silicoater, a number of studies have confirmed effective bonding of resin composites to Ni-Cr, Co-Cr, and titanium alloys.[37–41] Nevertheless, there are some potential problems in using this system, because thin edges of the restorations may be deformed and volume loss from precious metal alloys is much higher than from base metal alloys as a result of the high abrasion pressures.[38,42]

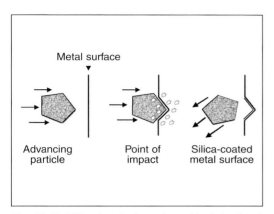

Fig 10-11 Tribochemical coating with Cojet-Sand (3M Espe).

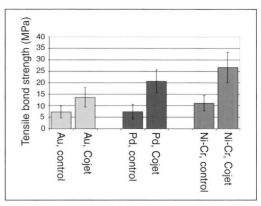

Fig 10-12 Tensile bond strength of Cojet-treated surfaces for gold, palladium, and Ni-Cr alloys bonded with Variolink II (Ivoclar Vivadent, Schaan, Liechtenstein).

A chairside coating system (Cojet, 3M Espe) has since been introduced for the resin bonding of metal-based crowns and fixed partial dentures and for the in situ repair of fractured metal-ceramic units with exposed metal surfaces. The technique for repair of fractured metal-ceramic restorations with exposed metal briefly involves the following steps:

1. Abrade the exposed metal surface with the intraoral abrasion instrument using the special particles provided.
2. Apply silane coupling agent.
3. Cover with opaquer and light cure.
4. Apply a layer of unfilled resin and light cure.
5. Complete repair with an esthetic resin composite.

As yet, little has been published to allow assessment of the effectiveness of this system to bond to precious metal alloys, but early results are encouraging.[43–45] Unpublished data from the University of Sheffield show a significant improvement in bond strength to both precious metal alloys and a Ni-Cr alloy (Fig 10-12).[46] However, these data also show that the improvement in the bond to the gold alloys was not as good as that to the palladium or Ni-Cr alloy.

One drawback with tribochemical coating is the need to purchase chairside equipment. The large number of steps involved also increases the potential for errors.

Metal Primers

What many clinicians would really like is a simple, inexpensive adhesive that they can apply directly to the metal surface using nothing more than a brush. The use of simple chemical pretreatment techniques of the alloy surface is therefore an area of increasing research. In particular, the use of coupling agents

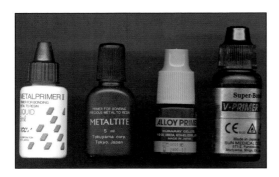

Fig 10-13 Commercially available metal primers for chairside and intraoral use.

Table 10-1 Commercially available metal primers

Product name	Primer	Manufacturer
V-Primer	VBATDT in 95% acetone	Sun Medical, Shiga, Japan
Alloy Primer	VBATDT/MDP	Kuraray, Osaka, Japan
Metal Primer II	MEPS in MMA	GC, Tokyo, Japan
Metaltite	MTU-6 in 96% ethanol	Tokuyama, San Mateo, CA

VBATDT = 6-(4-vinylbenzyl-n-propyl) amino-1,3,5-triazide-2,4-dithiol.
MDP = methacryloxyethyl-phenyl phosphate.
MEPS = methacryloyloxyalkyl thiophosphate derivatives.
MMA = methylmethacrylate.
MTU-6 = 6-methacryloyloxyhexyl 2-thiouracil-5-carboxylate.

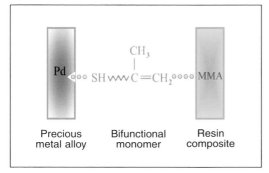

Fig 10-14 Schematic representation of a bifunctional monomer bonding a resin composite to a palladium alloy.

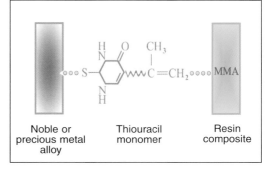

Fig 10-15 Structure and function of the Metaltite bifunctional monomer.

based on bifunctional monomers has gained interest because they have the potential to be effective yet simple alternatives to most of the surface modification techniques already described. They are usually supplied as single-liquid primers composed of a polymerizable monomer in a suitable solvent. A number of commercial products, based on these bifunctional primers, are now available (Fig 10-13 and Table 10-1). The products are invariably called primers despite the fact that they are coupling agents. The monomer has a bifunctional structure with one end carrying a methacryl or similar functional group for resin bonding and the other end carrying sulfur-containing groups for bonding to precious metal alloy (Fig 10-14). When the metal primer is applied to an airborne particle–abraded alloy surface, it is capable of enhanced adhesion to resin composites because of the ability of the mercapto groups to react with precious metal alloys and form a chemical bond.[47] Hence the presence of the mercapto groups allows chemical adhesion to precious metal alloy surfaces, as shown for a commercial product in Fig 10-15.

The product V-Primer is based on a bifunctional monomer that was first synthesized in 1987.[48] The bond strength and bond durability of luting resins in conjunction with this metal primer to a variety of precious metal alloys has been examined, and this product has been found to be particularly effective when used in conjunction with a 4-META–based resin.[49] However, the resin bond with V-Primer appears to be affected by the type of polymerization initiators used, and it would appear that resins using camphorquinone as the initiator should be avoided.[50,51] This is possibly due

to this bifunctional monomer having a vinyl end group as opposed to a methacrylate end group for bonding to the resin. This would seem to be confirmed by one study,[52,53] which found that the V-Primer improved bonding to base metal and precious metal alloys but that results were not consistently favorable for all alloy types (Fig 10-16). In contrast, the other metal primers did not appear to be resin specific and showed a significant improvement in bond strength to all alloy types, which confirms findings in other studies.[54–56] There is, however, still a question about the best combination of alloy, primer, and luting resin to use, as some combinations appear more hydrolytically stable than others.[57–59]

It would seem that for the moment it can be suggested that Metal Primer II and Metaltite combine well with composite and phosphonated luting resins, while V-Primer and Alloy Primer are best used with 4-META–based luting resins.

To make an intraoral repair rather than resin bond a restoration, one requirement is the placement of a thin layer of opaque resin to mask out the color of the underlying metal. The few studies evaluating this factor have been concerned with laboratory resins rather than the opaque resins available with resin composite restorative materials.[59–61] The optical opacifiers used in these resins are typically titania or zirconia. Unlike the aluminosilicate glasses used in resin composites, these fillers do not bond to the resin matrix via a silane coupling agent because these oxides are notoriously unreactive.[62] Yet, it is vital that some means of coating these opaque fillers is employed to ensure that the mechanical properties of the opaque resin are not compromised[63]; otherwise, fractures may recur after repair as a result of

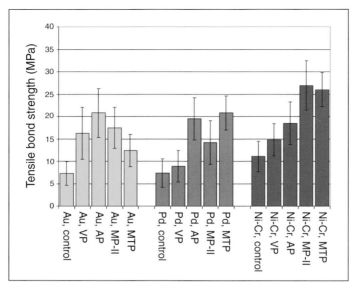

Fig 10-16 Tensile bond strengths for metal primers bonded to gold, palladium, and Ni-Cr alloys with Variolink II. (VP) V-Primer; (AP) Alloy Primer; (MP-II) Metal Primer II; (MTP) Metaltite.

cohesive failure of the opaque resin. More work is needed in this area to ensure that the resins used in intraoral repairs will be as effective as the luting resins. It has been shown that establishing a strong and durable bond between resin and precious metal alloys is possible, and it would be a shame if this were compromised by potentially poor mechanical properties of the opaque resin.

Conclusions

The increasing demand for clinical procedures involving resin-to-metal bonding has resulted in the development of a plethora of metal-bonding materials and procedures. Based on a personal interpretation of the evidence presented, the following recommendations are made:

For resin-bonded prostheses, a tough luting resin, such as C&B Superbond, will provide excellent bonding to the Ni-Cr alloy while also acting as a structural adhesive.

For the cementation of base metal crowns and fixed partial dentures, a phosphonated luting resin, such as Panavia 21, is preferred because of its excellent handling characteristics.

For the cementation of precious metal crowns and fixed partial dentures, the Cojet system in combination with a dual-cure luting resin is a reasonable and flexible option.

For intraoral repairs involving exposed metal, use of one of the metal primers compatible with conventional bis-GMA– and UDMA-based resin composites is a simple and low-cost solution.

References

1. Barzilay I, Myers ML, Cooper LB, Graser GN. Mechanical and chemical retention of laboratory cured composite to metal surfaces. J Prosthet Dent 1988;59:131–137.

2. Berge M. Properties of prosthetic resin-veneer materials processed in commercial laboratories. Dent Mater 1989;5:77–82.

3. Jones RM, Goodacre CJ, Moore BK, Dykema RW. A comparison of the physical properties of four prosthetic veneering materials. J Prosthet Dent 1989;61:38–44.

4. Jones RM, Moore BK, Goodacre CJ, Munoz-Viveros CA. Microleakage and shear bond strength of resin and porcelain veneers bonded to cast alloys. J Prosthet Dent 1991;65:221–228.

5. Rochette AL. Attachment of a splint to enamel of lower anterior teeth. J Prosthet Dent 1973; 30:418–423.

6. Saunders WP. Resin-bonded bridgework: A review. J Dent 1989;17:255–265.

7. Naegeli DG, Duke ES, Schwartz R, Norling BK. Adhesive bonding of composites to a casting alloy. J Prosthet Dent 1988;60:279–283.

8. Livaditis GJ. A chemical etching system for creating micromechanical retention in resin-bonded retainers. J Prosthet Dent 1986;56:181–188.

9. Livaditis GJ, Thompson VP. Etched castings: An improved retentive mechanism for resin-bonded retainers. J Prosthet Dent 1982;47:52–58.

10. Ózcan M, Pfeiffer P, Nergiz I. A brief history and current status of metal and ceramic surface conditioning concepts for resin bonding in dentistry. Quintessence Int 1998;29:713–724.

11. Kern N, Neikes MJ, Strub JR. Optimizing the bond between metal and bonding agent in bonded restorations using a simplified silicoating procedure. Dtsch Zahnartzl Z 1990;45:502–505.

12. Watanabe F, Powers LJ, Lorey RE. In vitro bonding of prosthodontic adhesives to dental alloys. J Dent Res 1988;67:479–483.

13. Atta M, Smith BGN, Brown D. Bond strength of three chemical adhesive cements adhered to nickel-chromium alloy for direct bonded retainers. J Prosthet Dent 1990;63:137–143.

14. Barclay CW, Williams R. The tensile and shear bond strength of a conventional and a 4-META self-cure acrylic resin to various surface finishes of Co-Cr alloy. Eur J Prosthodont Restor Dent 1994;3:5–9.

15. Jacobson TE. The significance of adhesive denture base resin. Int J Prosthodont 1989;2: 163–172.

16. Tanaka T, Nagata K, Takeyama M, Atsuta M, Nakabayashi N, Masuhara E. 4-META opaque resin—A new resin strongly adhesive to nickel-chromium alloy. J Dent Res 1981;60:1697–1702.

17. Creugers NHJ, Käyser AF. An analysis of multiple failures of resin-bonded bridges. J Dent 1992;20:348–351.

18. Degrange M, Attal J-P. Resin bonded to metal: Roughness, wettability, adhesion inter-relations [in French]. J Biomater Dent 1992;7:103–109.

19. Durkee MC, Thompson VP. [Letter.] Int J Prosthodont 1996;9:100–103.

20. Northeast SE, van Noort R, Shaglouf AS. Tensile peel failure of resin-bonded Ni/Cr beams: An experimental and finite element study. J Dent 1994;22:252–256.

21. Degrange M, Charrier JL, Attal J-P, Asmussen E. Bonding of luting materials for resin-bonded bridges: Clinical relevance of in vitro test. J Dent 1994;22(suppl 1):S28–S32.

22. McLean JW. A new method of bonding dental cements and porcelain to metal surfaces. Oper Dent 1977;2:130–142.

23. Ayad MF, Rosenstiel SF. Preliminary evaluation of tin plating for extracoronal restorations: Evaluation of marginal quality and retention. Int J Prosthodont 1998;11:44–48.

24. Gates WD, Diaz-Arnold AM, Aquilino SA, Ryther JS. Comparison of the adhesive strength of a BIS-GMA cement to tin-plated and non–tin-plated alloys. J Prosthet Dent 1993;69:12–16.

25. Rubo JH, Pegoraro LF, Ferreira PM. A comparison of tensile bond strengths of resin-retained prostheses made using five alloys. Int J Prosthodont 1996;9:277–281.

26. Rubo JH, Pegoraro LF, Marolato F, Rubo MH. The effect of tin-electroplating on the bond of four dental alloys to resin cement: An in vitro study. J Prosthet Dent 1998;80:27–31.

27. Kiatsirirote K, Northeast SE, van Noort R. Bonding procedures for intraoral repair of exposed metal with resin composite. J Adhes Dent 1999; 1:315–321.

28. Imbery TA, Davis RD. Evaluation of tin plating systems for a high-noble alloy. Int J Prosthodont 1993;6:55–60.

29. Tanaka T, Thompson VP. Evaluation of new bonding systems for non-oxidized noble alloys [abstract 1191]. J Dent Res 1992;71:254.

30. Vallittu PK. Bonding of hybrid composite resin to the surface of gold-alloy used in porcelain-fused-to-metal restorations. J Oral Rehabil 1997;24:560–567.

31. Laufer BZ, Nicholls JI, Townsend ID. SiO_X-C coating: A composite-to-metal bonding mechanism. J Prosthet Dent 1988;60:320–327.

32. Musil R, Garsschke A, Tiller HJ, Bimberg R. New aspects of synthetic resin-metal bonding in crown and bridge techniques. Dent Labor 1982;12:1711–1716.

33. Creugers NHJ, Welle PR, Vrijhoef MMA. Four bonding systems for resin-retained cast metal prostheses. Dent Mater 1988;4:85–88.

34. Kern M, Thompson VP. Influence of prolonged thermal cycling and water storage on the tensile bond strength of composite to Ni-Cr alloy. Dent Mater 1994;9:19–25.

35. Guggenberger R. Rocatec system—Adhesion by tribochemical coating. Dtsch Zahnartzl Z 1989;44:874–876.

36. Peutzfeldt A, Asmussen E. Silicoating: Evaluation of a new method of bonding composite resin to metal. Scand Dent J 1988;96:171–176.

37. Kern M, Thompson VP. Sandblasting and silica-coating of dental alloys: Volume loss, morphology and changes in the surface composition. Dent Mater 1993;9:155–161.

38. Kern M, Thompson VP. Effect of sandblasting and silica-coating procedures on pure titanium. J Dent 1994;22:300–306.

39. May KB, Fox J, Razzoog ME, Lang BR. Silane to enhance the bond between polymethyl methacrylate and titanium. J Prosthet Dent 1995;73:428–431.

40. Moulin P, Picard B, Degrange M. Water resistance of resin-bonded joints with time related to alloy surface treatment. J Dent 1999;27:79–87.

41. Nabadalung DP, Powers JM, Connelly ME. Comparison of bond strength of three denture base resins to treated nickel-chromium-beryllium alloy. J Prosthet Dent 1998;80:354–361.

42. Pröbster L, Kourtis S. Surface morphology of alloys treated with the Rocatec system. Dtsch Zahnartzl Z 1991;46:135–139.

43. Cob DS, Vargas MA, Fridrich TA, Bouschlicher MR. Metal surface treatment: Characterization and effect on composite-to-metal bond strength. Oper Dent 2000;25:427–433.

44. Frankenberger R, Krämer N, Sindel J. Repair strength of etched vs silica-coated metal—Ceramic and all-ceramic restorations. Oper Dent 2000;25:209–215.

45. Sun R, Suansuwan N, Kilpatrick N, Swain M. Characterisation of tribochemically assisted bonding of composite resin to porcelain and metal. J Dent 2000;28:441–445.

46. Manani AP, van Noort R. Novel adhesion promoters as metal primers for dental alloys [abstract 1824]. J Dent Res 2001;80:754.

47. Suzuki M, Fujishima A, Miyazaki T, Hisamitsu H, Kojima K, Kadoma Y. A study on the adsorption structure of an adhesive monomer for precious metals by surface-enhanced Raman scattering spectroscopy. Biomaterials 1999;20:839–845.

48. Kojima K, Kadoma Y, Imai Y. Adhesion to precious metals utilizing triazine dithione derivative monomer. Jpn J Dent Mater 1987;6:702–707.

49. Matsumura H, Kamada K, Tanoue N, Atsuta M. Effect of thione primers on bonding of noble metal alloys with an adhesive resin. J Dent 2000;28:287–293.

50. Yoshida K, Atsuta M. Effect of adhesive primers for noble metals on shear bond strengths of resin cements. J Dent 1997;25:53–58.

51. Yoshida K, Atsuta M. Effect of MMA-PMMA resin polymerization initiators on the bond strength of adhesive primers for noble metal. Dent Mater 1999;15:332–336.

52. El-Thwaini Y, Sudsangiam S, Northeast SE, van Noort R. The effectiveness of metal primers as adhesion promoters to a Au, Pd and Ni/Cr alloy [abstract 146]. J Dent Res 2000;79:162.

53. Sudsangiam S, van Noort R. The effectiveness of coupling agents as adhesion promoters to Au and Pd alloys [abstract 336]. J Dent Res 1999;78:147.

54. Antoniadou M, Kern M, Strub JR. Effect of a new metal primer on the bond strength between a resin cement and two high-noble alloys. J Prosthet Dent 2000;84:554–560.

55. Taira Y, Imai Y. Primer for bonding resin to metal. Dent Mater 1995;11:2–6.

56. Yoshida K, Kamada K, Sawase T, Atsuta M. Effect of three adhesive primers for noble metal on the shear bond strengths of three resin cements. J Oral Rehab 2001;28:14–19.

57. Atsuta M, Matsumura H, Tanaka T. Bonding fixed prosthodontic composite resin and precious metal alloys with the use of vinyl-thiol primer and an opaque resin. J Prosthet Dent 1992;67:296–300.

58. Matsumura H, Tanaka T, Atsuta M. Bonding of silver-palladium-copper-gold alloy with thiol derivative primers and tri-n-butylborane–initiated luting agents. J Oral Rehab 1997;24:291–296.

59. Yoshida K, Kamada K, Taira Y, Atsuta M. Effect of three adhesive primers on the bond strength of four light-activated opaque resins to noble alloy. J Oral Rehab 2001;28:168–173.

60. Ohkubo C, Watanabe I, Hosoi T, Okabe T. Shear bond strengths of polymethyl methacrylate to cast titanium and cobalt-chromium frameworks using five metal primers. J Prosthet Dent 2000;83:50–57.

61. Yoshida K, Taira Y, Sawase T, Atsuta M. Effects of adhesive primers on the bond strength of self-curing resin to cobalt-chromium alloy. J Prosthet Dent 1997;77:617–620.

62. Derand P, Derand T. Bond strength of luting cements to zirconium oxide ceramics. Int J Prosthodont 2000;13:131–135.

63. Yoshida K, Taira Y, Atsuta M. Properties of opaque resin composite containing coated and silanized titanium dioxide. J Dent Res 2001; 80:864–868.

Chapter 11

Adhesive Technologies and the Improved Quality of Delivered Dentistry

Ivar A. Mjör

Abstract

Adhesive technology in restorative dentistry has made major advances, but a great need exists for premarketing clinical testing of new and improved systems. Too many materials are introduced based on meager in vitro data, and too many materials disappear from the market within months after their introduction. Clinical testing must become the order of the day, or at least a postmarketing surveillance system must be established to assess the biologic side effects to the materials, among other factors. Practice-based studies should be included in this testing, despite the fact that they are hampered by many problems in interpreting the data.

Dentistry in the 21st century permits optimal esthetic reconstruction and replacement of diseased, defective, and lost teeth or parts of teeth. In fact, with the use of present adhesive techniques, an individual's esthetics can be improved by anatomic recontouring of malformed or malpositioned teeth and by closing unsightly diastemata. Adhesive dentistry has also expanded the field of restorative dentistry by allowing minimally invasive techniques to be employed for initial restorations and for repair of defects on existing restorations. Adhesive materials are also used in the prevention of caries by the application of pit and fissure sealants and in orthodontics to esthetically improve fixed appliances and at the same time secure them in place.

The present state of the art has taken almost 50 years to reach. With few exceptions, trial and error has been the main basis for the advances made in dental adhesive technology. This approach has largely been at the patients' expense. The optimism of manufacturers, clinicians, and patients toward the steady stream of new and improved products has at times not come to fruition, more often with regard to the longevity and cost effectiveness of resin composite restorations than due to disappointments in the esthetic result.

Brief History

After working with silicate cement as the only available tooth-colored restorative material for Class III and Class V restorations for decades, the dental profession was ready for a change, and preferably a change that allowed expanded use of tooth-colored restorative materials. Clinicians had reached the stage at which they were willing to accept any change as a change for the better. This attitude resulted in the marketing of cold-curing unfilled resins as esthetic restorative materials in the late 1940s. The experience with these nonadhesive tooth-colored materials became a tragedy for restorative dentistry. Many pulps became necrotic, and periapical abscesses developed, with endodontics and extraction as the final alternative treatments. This tragedy, however, had a positive side: It focused attention on the need for premarketing clinical and biological testing of restorative materials. The long road to establish standards for biologic testing began in the 1960s, and after years of discussion, methods for toxicity testing were established.[1]

Development of Resin Composites

A major event in the development of direct tooth-colored restorative materials was the introduction of the enamel acid-etch technique,[2] followed by the development of resin composite materials, a combination of dimethacrylate monomers and inorganic filler particles.[3] The introduction of these materials was accompanied by numerous investigations related to their properties, including biologic and clinical assessments. The biologic effects received particular attention at this time; in particular, possible adverse effects of acid etching of enamel,

and later of all of the mineralized dental tissues, were of great concern to many clinicians.[4] Somewhat controversial results were presented in these studies, but the introduction of the total-etch technique,[5] supported by solid clinical experience, has shown that acid etching of enamel, dentin, and cementum is biologically acceptable.

Excellent clinical results can be achieved with present-day direct resin composite materials, but optimal results require meticulous attention to details during placement of the restorations. The materials are technique sensitive, and it has become more important than ever to follow manufacturers' instructions for use of the materials. A number of improvements have been and are being presented, including development of simple clinical techniques. Despite the different structure and composition of enamel, dentin, and cementum, the goal is to treat these tissues the same way and still obtain optimal bonding. Four-, three-, two-, and one-bottle systems have been used to bond the materials to the dental substrates. These constant changes mean that this field of restorative dentistry is in a state of flux.

It is important to keep in mind that the main reason for the frequent changes in materials and techniques related to composite restorations is simply that the materials and techniques in present use are not good enough and have potential for improvement. The frequent introduction of new materials of a specific type may be looked upon as a sign of progress, but it may also be a sign of weakness. It seems that the quality of any group of materials at a given time is inversely related to the number of new products entering the market. Fifteen years ago a large number of resin composites entered the market. The number of new composites presently being introduced is low, but new bonding materials are introduced rather frequently. The situation reflects a stabilization of the quality of resin composites but uncertainty related to the quality of bonding agents.

It is also important in this context to realize that clinical evaluation and biologic testing are rarely carried out to support claims by manufacturers. The improvements in bonding are, at best, based on interpretation of laboratory tests done on poorly defined substrates. The lack of clinical testing is astounding, especially because the quality of the treatment is not monitored by any kind of formal postmarketing surveillance system. It is up to the dental profession as a whole to point out the need for both pre- and postmarketing evaluations and to be actively engaged in developing relevant programs. If routines for such evaluations are not established, engagements by third-party payment institutions and/or consumer associations may take a leading role in controlling the use of restorative materials.

Alternative Adhesive Materials

Glass-ionomer restorative materials were introduced in the early 1970s.[6] They bond to mineralized tissues and release fluoride. The first marketed materials had poor esthetics, and glass ionomers came into disrepute as an esthetically unacceptable tooth-colored alternative material. Their caries preventive effect has also been questioned.[7]

The traditional glass-ionomer restorative materials are still on the market, but resin-modified glass-ionomer materials and resin composites with fluoride-leaching glass fillers, the so-called compomers, have been introduced. They are easier to handle clinically, and to a large extent they have taken over the market share of glass ionomers.

This chapter will concentrate on the most commonly used tooth-colored direct restorative materials, resin composites, and they will be treated as a group of materials, even though materials with widely different properties are covered under the umbrella of the term. The advantage of using an indirect technique is that the anatomy of the restorations, including the contact points, can be better controlled, and the curing is enhanced. However, the slight advantages over a directly placed resin restoration can hardly justify the increased cost. Furthermore, resin-based luting cements have become an integral part of ceramic restorative technology and also for cementation of metal restorations. Special resin-based materials for indirect restorations are also available, both for traditional laboratory-prepared restorations and for the direct-indirect technique, by which the restoration is prepared in the mouth and partly cured, followed by a heat cure prior to cementation.

Clinical Testing of Restorative Materials

New dental restorative materials are traditionally tested according to the guidelines for the controlled clinical trials. The guidelines define the conditions for the testing, including the type of restoration to be placed, inclusion and exclusion criteria for patient selection (and they are often dental students or dental school staff), defined size of the restoration, and a number of other criteria. It does not specify the qualifications of the clinician placing the restorations, but often the clinician recognized as the most competent, and often with specialty training at a dental school, places the restorations. The selected clinician works with dental assistants and with no time constraints. Whether it takes 15 minutes or 2 hours to place a restoration is of no consequence, and meticulous finishing at a subsequent visit is part of the procedure. The clinical team has also read the instructions for use of the material, and team members have often practiced using the materials. Technique sensitivity is, therefore, rarely noted as a problem. Calibrated clinicians evaluate the results at predetermined intervals.

Practice-Based Research

The conditions for the controlled clinical trial are very different from those in an average general dental practice. No calibration of clinicians exists, and clinicians must rely on what they were taught in dental school (where calibration exercises are uncommon) or in continuing dental education courses (where clinical exercises are rarely included). The clinicians must rely on their clinical experience, whatever it encompasses. Obviously, scientific criteria cannot be met, because treatment in general dental practice inevitably involves many uncontrollable factors—including variations in

clinicians' treatment decisions, their sense of quality, their perception of what extent of defects constitutes a failure, the potential misunderstanding of definitions and instructions, and how they account for drop-out of patients—just to list a few of the variables. However, data from general dental practice have the decided advantage that they represent everyday, real-life dentistry, ie, the treatment the public at large receives. The present discussion will, therefore, focus on practice-based data.

Results from practice-based studies have repeatedly shown that the clinical diagnosis of secondary (recurrent) caries is by far the most common reason for replacement of all types of directly placed restorations, including resin-based– and glass-ionomer–type restorations.[8] This is different from the results obtained from controlled clinical trials.[9]

It is the view of the author that practice-based data are more clinically relevant than data from controlled clinical trials, despite the inherent problems with the scientific merit of the results. Reports on large numbers of restorations placed and replaced by a large number of clinicians may average out the subjectivity of the individual and provide a more relevant assessment of restorative materials than the results from the clinically artificial conditions of the controlled clinical trial.

Reasons for Failure of Adhesive Restorations

The reasons for replacement of resin composite restorations in general dental practice have changed markedly over the

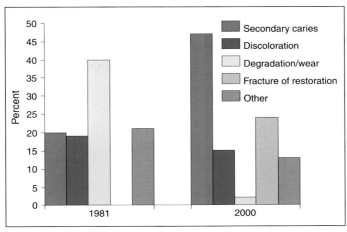

Fig 11-1 Reasons for replacements of resin composite restorations in permanent teeth of adults as recorded in general dental practice in 1981[10] and 2000.[11]

last 20 years (Fig 11-1), while those for amalgam have remained much the same.[7,10,12] Material degradation, often referred to as *wear*, of the restorations was a major problem with the composites that first entered the market.[13] It was primarily chemical erosion in vivo of inferior materials, accelerated by normal mastication. Marginal staining of resin composite restorations was also a common reason for failure of these restorations. This problem was probably associated with the hesitation by clinicians to acid etch the preparations. Bulk discoloration was another problem, and it reflected the poor chemical and physical properties of the materials.

The most recent practice-based data on resin composite restorations[11,14–18] indicate that apart from the clinical diagnosis of secondary caries, which covers almost half of all replaced restorations,

bulk and marginal fractures comprise about 25% of all reasons for clinically diagnosed failures. Bulk and marginal discoloration of composite restorations involve about 10% to 15% and tooth fracture about 5% to 10% of all restorations replaced. Thus, the reasons for clinically diagnosed failures of present-day resin composite restorations have become similar to those for amalgam restorations with the exception of discoloration, which is not an applicable criterion for metal restorations.

In discussions of reasons for failure of resin-based restorations, it is important to point out that the materials used seem to promote bacterial adhesion.[1,19] Optimal oral hygiene, including plaque control, is therefore of the utmost importance to maintain the restorations.

It is noteworthy that the reasons for replacement of the glass-ionomer materials

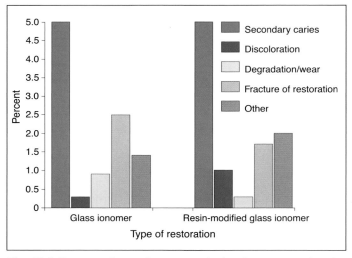

Fig 11-2 Reasons for replacement of glass-ionomer and resin-modified glass-ionomer restorations in general dental practice. Based on data from Mjör et al.[11]

are similar to those for the present-day composite (Fig 11-2) and amalgam restorations. About half of all restorations that are replaced have the clinical diagnosis of secondary caries, while bulk fracture of restorations is slightly more common for traditional glass-ionomer restorations than for resin-modified types. Thus, no apparent benefit of the fluoride release from the glass-ionomer materials can be recorded, although the patient selection may be different for this type of restoration. However, since the universal use of fluoride dentifrice is in effect, it is unlikely that the minimal release of fluoride from glass-ionomer restorations will have an additional beneficial effect beyond that from fluoride topically applied from dentifrice twice a day, which exceeds the leachable fluoride concentration of glass-ionomer materials by up to 1000 times.

Biological Side Effects

Toxic side effects of dental materials in general are rare,[20] but allergic reactions to a number of materials, including resin composites, have been reported. Adverse Reaction Units for Dental Materials have been established in Norway and Sweden as a postmarketing surveillance system to collect information and give advice to clinicians and patients about adverse reactions to dental materials.

Resin-based materials contain a number of potential toxic and allergenic components. Several different reactions to these materials have been reported. Occupational contact dermatitis is a problem for members of the dental team handling these materials.[21] In patients, skin rashes are the most common reaction. Asthmatic reactions also may occur.

Longevity and Cost-Benefit Effectiveness

The cost-benefit effectiveness of alternative restorative treatments can be estimated on the basis of two factors: (1) the initial cost of placing restorations and (2) the length of time the restorations last.[20] The cost for replacement of any type of tooth-colored restoration with the same material is often the same as that for the initial restoration, plus any fee adjustment for inflation. Therefore, longevity becomes the most important factor in deciding which alternative is most cost effective.

The longevity of restorations in practice-based studies are usually recorded as their age at replacement. In the typical cross-sectional study involving hundreds of replacements, a full range of ages of replaced restorations are found. The longevity is then expressed as the median value, or the time at which half of the restorations have been replaced. This "half life" value as an expression of longevity of a large number of failed restorations is particularly useful, because it eliminates the effect of outlier values, ie, values that deviate markedly from the mean.

The median age of replaced composite restorations increased in the late 1990s. In a review of reports from practice-based studies of restorations placed up until the late 1980s, the median age of composite restorations was about 4 years for large restorations.[22] In a Danish survey from 1987 to 1988[23] the median longevity of composite restorations was 6 years, and it had remained the same since a similar Danish survey from 1980 to 1982[24]

and a survey from Sweden in 1978 to 1979.[10] In a recent large study from Norway[7] the median age of replaced composite restorations was 8 years, the same as that from a small survey in Florida.[4] The recorded increase in longevity of composite restorations over the last 15 years may be attributed to a variety of reasons, with enhanced quality of the materials undoubtedly being one important factor.

It is also difficult to evaluate the impact of the slow introduction or lack of teaching of posterior composites in North American[25] and European[26] dental schools. The inconsistent teaching of cariology in some parts of the world is also a problem for restorative dentistry in general. The clinical diagnosis "secondary caries," for example, inevitably leads to replacement of the entire restoration. A survey of the teaching of criteria for secondary caries in North American dental schools[27] leaves much to be desired in the definition and practical implication of this clinical diagnosis.

It should also be pointed out that the type (Fig 11-3) and size of the restoration are factors in determining the longevity of restorations, and that the larger the composite restoration, the lower its age at failure. An increase in the proportion of posterior composite restorations has occurred during the last 10 years. Therefore, the overall median age of composite restorations of 8 years is not directly comparable to the 6 years referred to above when Class III and Class V were the predominant composite restorations; rather, it represents an underestimation of the age of small or one-surface restorations. At present, resin composite materials are used as universal restora-

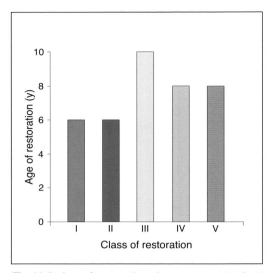

Fig 11-3 Age of restorations in permanent teeth at the time of replacement in general dental practice. Based on data from Mjör et al.[7]

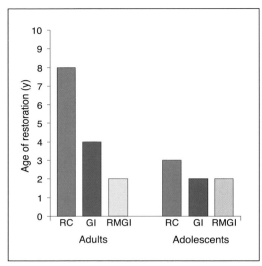

Fig 11-4 Age of resin composite (RC), glass-ionomer (GI) and resin-modified glass-ionomer (RMGI) restorations in adults (≥ 19 y) and adolescents (≤ 18 y) at the time of replacement in general dental practice. Based on data from Mjör et al.[7]

tive materials for all classes of restorations by clinicians in many countries.

A number of other factors have been shown to affect the longevity of restorations: for example, whether primary or permanent teeth are studied.[23] The age of replaced restorations in the permanent teeth of adolescents is much lower than that in adults (Fig 11-4).[7,23] Patient factors such as oral hygiene,[28] as well as the method of remuneration for the treatment, may also play a role.[29] It has further been shown that the clinician's years in practice affects the age of restorations at replacement. The restorations replaced by a more experienced clinician are, in general, older than those replaced by less experienced clinicians.[7] The more experienced clinician also diagnoses fewer cases of secondary caries than do clinicians with less clinical experience.[14]

Repair of Restorations

Several diagnoses of failures of restorations are subjective and ill defined, notably secondary caries, which is the most frequent reason for replacement of restorations. In a recent review of secondary caries as a clinical diagnosis, it was pointed out that its development was not related to microleakage or to the size of the crevice at the tooth-restoration interface, but that it developed the same way as primary caries lesions, ie, from the external surface inward.[30] Since secondary caries usually is a localized defect, it may lend itself to repair rather than total replacement of the restoration, provided that access can be gained and the restoration otherwise is serviceable. By removing enough of the restorative material adjacent to the lesion, the extent of the caries lesion and the possibility of removing it completely can be assessed. If the lesion is limited in extent, repair of the defect should always be considered. Similarly, margin fracture of composite restorations may be repaired rather than result in replacement of the restoration. Surface finishing of unsightly composite restorations also allows a differentiation between bulk discoloration and surface staining, the latter being easily remedied by polishing. Such approaches are often feasible, as well as minimally invasive. However, there is a lack of published longevity data or other outcome measurements, although such research programs are in progress (Gordan and collaborators, personal communication, 2001).

Conclusions

The esthetics of dental restorative treatment has become an important part of patients' evaluation of treatment quality. Adhesive technology plays an important part in the drive toward optimal esthetics. The longevity of the treatment has become second to esthetics in the evaluation of quality among patients in industrialized countries.

Acknowledgment

A Guest Research Fellowship from the Research Council of Norway as a supplement to the author's Faculty Developmental Leave is gratefully acknowledged.

References

1. Skjørland KK. Plaque accumulation on different dental filling materials. Scand J Dent Res 1973; 81:538–542.
2. Buonocore MB. A simple method of increasing the adhesion of acrylic filling materials to enamel surfaces. J Dent Res 1955;35:846–851.
3. Bowen RL [inventor]. Dental filling material comprising vinyl silane treatment fused silica and a binder consisting of the reaction product of BIS phenol and glycidyl acrylate. US patent 3,066,112. 1962.
4. Mjör IA, Moorhead J. Selection of restorative materials, reasons for replacement and longevity of restorations in Florida. J Am Coll Dent 1998;65:27–33.
5. Fusayama T. New Concepts in Operative Dentistry. Tokyo: Quintessence, 1980:118–119.
6. Wilson AD, Kent BE. A new translucent cement for dentistry. The glass ionomer cement. Br Dent J 1972;132:133–135.
7. Mjör IA, Dahl JE, Moorhead JE. The age of restorations at placement in permanent teeth in general dental practice. Acta Odontol Scand 2000;58:97–101.
8. Deligeorgi V, Mjör IA, Wilson NHF. An overview of reasons for the placement and replacement of restorations. Prim Dent Care 2001;8:5–11.
9. Mjör IA. The basis for everyday, real-life operative dentistry. Oper Dent 2001;26:521–524.
10. Mjör IA. Placement and replacement of restorations. Oper Dent 1981;6:49–54.
11. Mjör IA, Moorhead JE, Dahl JE. Reasons for replacement of restorations in permanent teeth in general dental practice. Int Dent J 2000;50: 360–366.
12. Mjör IA. Direct posterior filling materials. In: Vanherle G, Degrange M, Willems G (eds). State-of-the-Art on Direct Posterior Filling Materials and Dentine Bonding. Leuven, Belgium: van der Poorten, 1993:1–13.
13. Ruyter IE. Monomer systems and polymerization. In: Vanherle G, Smith DC (eds). Posterior Composite Resin Dental Restorative Materials. Utrecht, The Netherlands: Peter Szulc, 1985: 109–135.

14. Mjör IA, Shen C, Eliasson ST, Richter S. Placement and replacement of restorations in general dental practice in Iceland. Oper Dent 2002; 27:117–123.

15. Wilson NA, Whitehead SA, Mjör IA, Wilson NH. Reasons for the placement and replacement of crowns in general dental practice. Prim Dent Care 2003;10:53–59.

16. Mjör IA, Gordan WV. Failure, repair, refurbishing and longevity of restorations. Oper Dent 2002;27:528–534.

17. Burke FJ, Wilson NH, Cheung SW, Mjör IA. Influence of the method of funding on the age of failed restorations in general dental practice in the UK. Br Dent J 2002;192:699–702.

18. Mjör IA, Shen C, Eliasson ST, Richter S. Placement and replacement of restorations in general dental practice in Iceland. Oper Dent 2002; 27:117–123.

19. Svanberg M, Mjör IA, Ørstavik D. Mutans streptococci in plaque from margins of amalgam, composite and glass-ionomer restorations. J Dent Res 1990;68:861–864.

20. Mjör IA. Problems and benefits associated with restorative materials. Side effects and cost-benefit analysis. Adv Dent Res 1992;6:7–16.

21. Hensten-Pettersen A, Jacobsen N. Biocompatibility of restorative materials. Oper Dent 2001;(suppl 6):229–235.

22. Mjör IA, Jokstad A, Qvist V. Longevity of posterior restorations. Int Dent J 1990;40:11–17.

23. Qvist V, Qvist J, Mjör IA. Placement and longevity of tooth-colored restorations in Denmark. Acta Odontol Scand 1990;48:305–311.

24. Qvist V, Thylstrup A, Mjör IA. Restorative treatment pattern and longevity of resin restorations in Denmark. Acta Odontol Scand 1986;44:351–356.

25. Mjör IA, Wilson NHF. The teaching of Class I and Class II direct composite restorations in North American dental schools. J Am Dent Assoc 1998;129:1415–1421.

26. Wilson NHF, Mjör IA. The teaching of Class I and Class II direct composite restorations in European dental schools. J Dent 2000;28:15–21.

27. Clark TD, Mjör IA. Current teaching of cariology in North American dental schools. Oper Dent 2001;26:412–418.

28. Burke FJT, Wilson NHF, Cheung SW, Mjör IA. Influence of patient factors on age of restorations at failure and reasons for their placement and replacement. J Dent 2001;29:317–324.

29. Burke FJT, Wilson NHF, Cheung SW, Mjör IA. Influence of the method of funding on the age of failed restorations in general dental practice in the UK. Br Dent J 2002;192:699–702.

30. Mjör IA, Toffenetti F. Secondary caries: A literature review with case reports. Quintessence Int 2000;31:165–179.

Chapter 12

Can Technology Cure Disease?

Jean-François Roulet, Stefan Zimmer

Abstract

Caries, like periodontal disease, creates spectacular tissue destruction. Since the early days of dentistry, dentists have believed that they could cure caries by eliminating the destroyed tissue and replacing it with restorations. This belief has triggered the development of many outstanding technologies to restore teeth. But as valuable as these techniques are, they do nothing to cure the disease; they only treat the symptoms. Curing a disease means eliminating its causes, and clinicians must be intent on this goal. Restorative dentists must do more to fight caries and periodontitis than simply implement preventive measures. For instance, by designing reconstructions in such a way that all plaque retention sites are eliminated or are easily cleanable, the risk for plaque to be reestablished is greatly decreased. Also, the use of adhesive techniques virtu-ally eliminates every marginal gap, thus rendering recurrent caries an unlikely event. Technology can contribute to the elimination of disease, but only biotechnology will be able to cure caries and periodontitis.

It is a worldwide misconception that caries can be treated with restorations. Doing this, within seconds the clinician destroys with the high-speed handpiece more sound hard tissue than the caries destroyed in months or even years. If clinicians follow the principles of G. V. Black for the preparation of cavities, this effect is even more pronounced. Since with restorative therapy only the symptom of caries (the decayed tissue) is eliminated, it is only a matter of time until the caries recurs. This is called *recurrent caries* (Fig 12-1). Clinicians believe that use of good materials (eg, gold) will increase the suc-

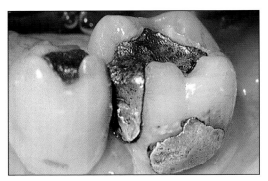

Fig 12-1 Amalgam restoration with recurrent caries.

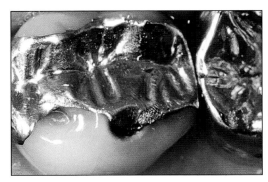

Fig 12-2 Gold inlay with recurrent caries.

Table 12-1 Replacement of restorations*

Author	Country	No. of restorations	Material	(%) replacements
Mjör (1981)	Norway	5187	amalgam	71
Mjör (1981)	Norway	5187	tooth-colored	79
Klausner et al (1987)	USA	5511	–	54

*Based on data from Mjör[1] and Klausner et al.[2]

cess and the longevity of a restoration. Unfortunately, this is not true, because this does not treat the cause of caries. As long as the situation remains unchanged, caries will still be present at the predilection sites—restoration margins, to name one (Fig 12-2). As a result, most restorations are replacements of other restorations,[1,2] and the most frequent reason for replacement indicated by clinicians in surveys is caries (Table 12-1).

This approach has triggered the development of more sophisticated technology for restorative dentistry: Air rotor, micromotor, silicone impression materials, porcelain-fused-to-metal restorations, all-ceramic crowns, resin composites, adhesive technology, and use of computer-aided design/computer-assisted manufacture technology are impressive milestones in restorative dentistry. But unfortunately, despite the technological progress, the basic concept has not changed and is no different from that of "dental therapists" in developing countries who extract teeth and manufacture simple dentures.

The combination of a "restorative" clinical approach with the systems of remuneration that pay for restorations (price per item) worldwide had fatal consequences. Despite the knowledge of the etiology of caries and periodontal diseases, which inherently gives clinicians

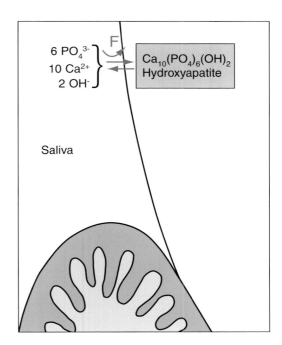

$$6 \ PO_4^{3-}$$
$$10 \ Ca^{2+} \quad \rightleftharpoons \quad Ca_{10}(PO_4)_6(OH)_2$$
$$2 \ OH^-$$

F

Hydroxyapatite

Saliva

Fig 12-3 Fluoride is entering the equilibrium between remineralization and demineralization, favoring the former by decreasing the critical pH for demineralization and acting as a "biocatalyst."

the keys for prevention, applied dentistry was driven into the "restorative track," with the consequences of extremely high expenditures for dentistry and probably overtreatment of patients. In Germany more money is spent treating the consequences of caries than treating heart and coronary diseases—both of which are diet-related. (In 1999, 20.2 billion DM were spent treating caries, compared with 15.4 billion DM spent treating heart and circulatory diseases.)

The Cure: Causal Therapy

The key is to understand the etiology of caries.[3,4] Based on the concept of a multi-factorial disease, basic principles of caries prevention can be formulated:

- Fight the microorganisms
- Decrease the frequency of sugar intake
- Apply fluorides

The first two measures are targeted at a cause of the caries. Therefore, it can be concluded that prevention is causal therapy, which is the best that medicine can offer. Fluoridation is an effective causal therapy. It cannot eliminate the causes, but by influencing the process of demineralization and remineralization (Fig 12-3), it can prevent the initial disease in its basic etiologic mechanism, which is far better than merely eliminating the symptoms.

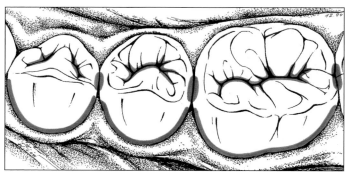

Fig 12-4 The predilection sites for caries.

The Contribution of Technology

Knowing the important factors in the etiology of caries, the clinician can apply technology and professional skills to benefit the patient's oral health with causal therapy. One etiologic factor for caries is microbial plaque. Based on the knowledge that microorganisms colonize on teeth wherever there are sheltered niches, the clinician can deduce the predilection sites for caries (Fig 12-4). On the other hand, it is the duty of the clinician to avoid the creation of any retention sites for microorganisms. The following rules can be postulated:

- Avoid overhangs of direct restorations by using an appropriate matrix band technique with careful wedging (eg, sectional matrices for posterior composites).
- Avoid the occurrence of marginal openings by using a precise adhesive technique with direct composite restorations as well as indirect composite or ceramic restorations.

- Avoid overhangs with all fixed partial dentures with the use of an accurate impression and laboratory technique.
- Make all interproximal areas cleanable for the patient (use of floss or an interdental brush).
- Knowing that margins of restorations are preferred sites of plaque retention, place them in areas that are readily accessible with a patient's cleaning techniques.
- Do not place finish lines subgingivally. If the decay has progressed into this area, it is better to perform a crown-lengthening procedure prior to restoration (Fig 12-5).

With knowledge of caries etiology, one could conclude that a clean tooth can never decay. However, it is known that oral hygiene measures alone cannot prevent caries.[5,6] Furthermore, it is difficult to completely remove plaque from a dentition. Therefore, technology can help here also, by improving the design of toothbrushes to increase their effectiveness.

One study[7] compared the Superbrush (Denta, Minde/Bergen, Norway) (Fig 12-6)

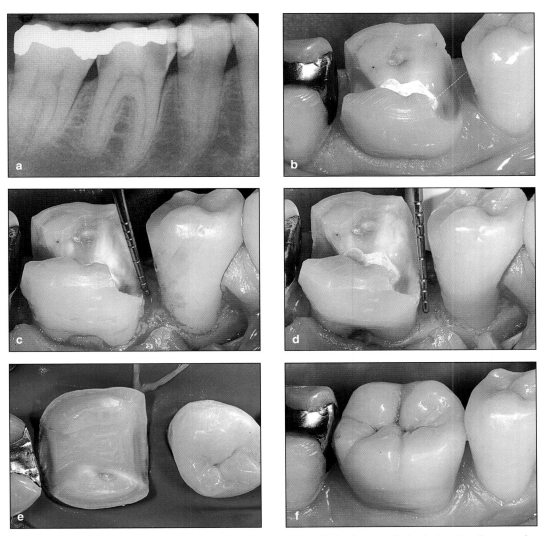

Figs 12-5a to 12-5f Crown-lengthening procedure to prevent placing a subgingival restorative margin. (Courtesy of Dr Roberto Spreafico.)

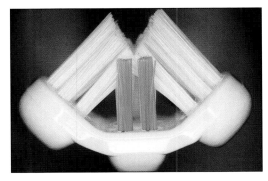

Fig 12-6 Superbrush.

Table 12-2 The effect of brushing with three different toothbrushes on plaque removal and gingival health*

Indices by age groups

	Plaque index (Quigley-Hein)			Papillary bleeding index (Mühlemann)		
	E39	PC	SB	E39	PC	SB
Children (6–12 y, n = 12)	2.25	2.12	1.39	0.41	0.40	0.30
Students (23–35 y, n = 12)	1.19	1.31	0.62	0.57	0.52	0.29
Adults (37–60 y, n = 12)	1.55	1.44	0.81	0.67	0.65	0.43

*Medians of the Quigley-Hein plaque index and the papillary bleeding index at the end of the study. The horizontal bars connect significantly different values at $P < .05$. (From Zimmer et al 1999.[7])
E39 = conventional manual toothbrush
PC = Powered toothbrush
SB =Superbrush (see Fig 12-6)

with a powered toothbrush (Braun-Oral B D 5525, Braun, Frankfurt/Main, Germany) and a conventional manual toothbrush (Elmex Super 29 and 39, respectively; GABA, Lörrach, Germany). Using a randomized crossover design with three age groups of test subjects, the results showed that the Superbrush was significantly superior to the other brushes (Table 12-2). Another study demonstrated the effectiveness of powered toothbrushes working in the sonic range.[8] Sonicare (Philips, Hamburg, Germany) and Water Pik Sonic Speed (Teledyne Water Pik, Fort Collins, CO) were compared with a manual toothbrush. The results clearly showed the superiority of the powered brushes (Figs 12-7a to 12-7c).

The other important factor in caries etiology is the substrate: sugar. Theoretically the rule "no sugar, no caries" is true; however, there is no need to completely ban

sugar. With the knowledge of the local mechanisms of decalcification, one can deduce a more clever strategy. It is known from plaque telemetry[9] that whenever plaque is confronted with sugar, the substrate will be metabolized into organic acids (mainly lactate), which decrease the local pH dramatically (Fig 12-8). If the pH drops below 5.7 (critical pH), hydroxyapatite will be dissolved (demineralization). After a certain amount of time (about 30 minutes), the sugar is metabolized and the acid production decreases, resulting in increasing pH. Since the ions are trapped in the plaque within a solution, they cannot maintain this status because of the solubility product, which is pH dependent. Therefore, they return into the crystalline lattice of the enamel (remineralization). However, if a pH drop occurs too often, the demineralization phase by far exceeds the remineralization, and the

Figs 12-7a to 12-7c Comparison of two powered toothbrushes (Sonic Speed and Sonicare) with a manual toothbrush (Elmex Sensitive). (For each group, n = 36.)

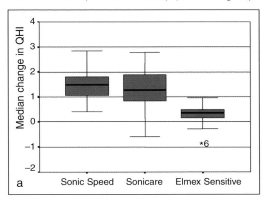

a

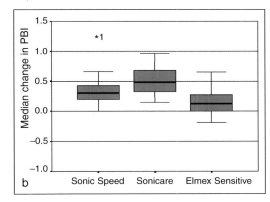

b

Fig 12-7a Changes in Quigley-Hein index (QHI).

Fig 12-7b Changes in modified papillary bleeding index (PBI).

Fig 12-7c Changes in approximal plaque index (API).

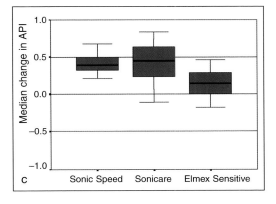

c

Fig 12-8 Plaque-pH telemetry after 4 days of abstinence from oral hygiene. As soon as plaque is confronted with sucrose (6), the pH drops dramatically and remains low for a substantial amount of time. Enamel demineralization starts at a pH of 5.7. In contrast, this does not occur when a tooth-friendly lozenge containing noncariogenic sugar substitutes is sucked (2). (Courtesy of Prof Dr Lutz Stoesser, University of Jena, Germany)

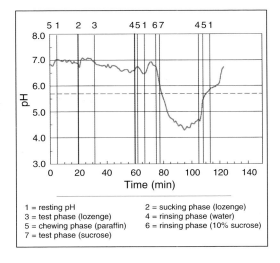

1 = resting pH
2 = sucking phase (lozenge)
3 = test phase (lozenge)
4 = rinsing phase (water)
5 = chewing phase (paraffin)
6 = rinsing phase (10% sucrose)
7 = test phase (sucrose)

187

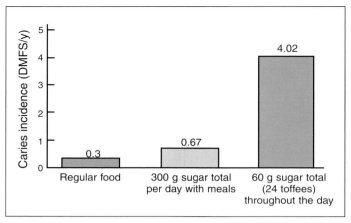

Fig 12-9 Frequent sugar ingestion yields extremely high caries incidence. (DMFS = decayed, missing, or filled surfaces.) (Data taken from Gustafsson et al.[10])

first result is a subsurface lesion, which develops into a larger lesion. The practical application of this theoretical knowledge is to recommend sugar-free snacks between meals and to restrict sugar consumption to the main meals, thus reducing the acid attacks to the enamel to a few episodes per day. This allows enough time for repair (remineralization).

These theories were proven in an in vivo study in which patients were subjected to different sugar ingestion regimens.[10] The caries incidence doubled in patients who were given 300 g of sugar per day, consumed only with main meals. By comparison, the test group, who consumed 60 g of sugar per day in the form of 24 toffees every day, had 15 times more caries than the control group (Fig 12-9). Some "tooth-friendly" sweets, including a chocolate, have been devel-

oped so that the pH under the plaque will not drop below 5.7 when the snack is eaten.

The last factor in caries prevention is the use of fluorides. Technology can help to produce efficient fluoride varnishes that have a good retention to the teeth and act as a slow release agent for fluoride. With this type of product, the beneficial effect of fluoride can be maintained for a long time, because a long-lasting fluoride reservoir can develop under the varnish.

Furthermore, adhesive technology is also helping to reduce the incidence of recurrent caries. Some excellent and effective adhesives are available that completely seal the dentin and produce gap-free restorations (Fig 12-10).[11] Bonded ceramic inlays have proven to maintain this seal in vivo for many years (Fig 12-11).[12]

Fig 12-10 Margin qualities in dentin of Class V restorations placed with different adhesives. Margin quality is determined by the percentage of continuous margin in the total margin length in dentin ($P > .05$). The statistical evaluation (vertical line for all products for which the difference in results is not statistically significant) is performed in comparison to the results of Syntac Classic and Optibond FL, the so-called gold standards of these materials. (Courtesy of Dr Uwe Blunck.)

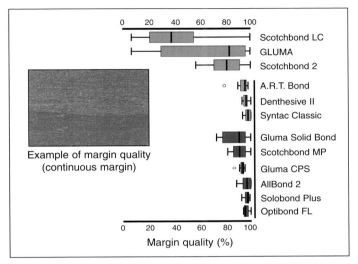

Fig 12-10a Adhesives of the first generations (orange), dentin conditioning adhesive systems (light green) and multi-step total-etch adhesive systems (dark green).

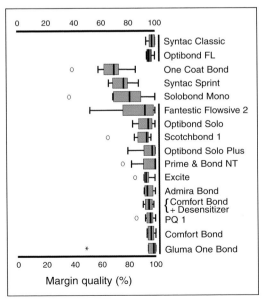

Fig 12-10b Total-etch one-step adhesive systems (blue) and gold standard (green).

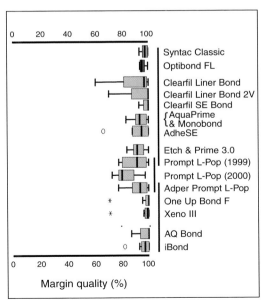

Fig 12-10c Self-etching adhesive systems (blue) and gold standard (green).

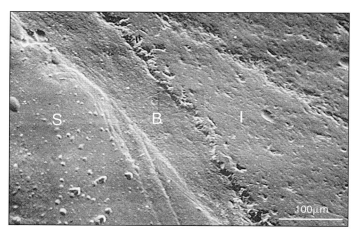

Fig 12-11 Portion of an adhesively luted ceramic inlay after 6 years in service. Marginal gaps are absent. (S = enamel; B = luting composite; I = inlay.) (From Kanzler and Roulet.[12])

A Treatment Concept

The treatment concept is based on two principles:

1. Do the causal therapy first. Only then may the restoration be done.
2. Prevention is the philosophical base of the concept. This means that the first question to ask when treating a patient is, "What must be done to prevent further disease?"

Treatment to satisfy the patient's demands regarding esthetics and chewing comfort must be done in a healthy mouth.

The concept can be divided into four phases[13]:

1. *The systemic phase, or diagnostics:* The objective of this phase is to fully understand the patient. The more knowledge acquired, the better. Thorough diagnostics minimizes the treatment risk. The final outcome of this phase is a treatment plan, which must be discussed with the patient.
2. *The hygiene phase, or elimination of the causes of the disease:* This is the most important phase in the treatment, because it is the causal therapy. Most of it can be delegated to a dental hygienist. It is the duty of the clinician during this phase to enable the patient to comply with oral hygiene expectations; ie, for the patient to achieve optimal cleaning, all overhangs, as well as all active caries sites, must be eliminated. This is usually done with semipermanent restorations, eg, glass-ionomer cement restorations or high-quality provisional fixed partial dentures (metal base with resin veneers).
3. *The corrective phase:* This phase is usually known as therapy. Only after the disease has been treated during the hygiene phase can the permanent restorations be made according to the treatment plan.
4. *The maintenance phase:* This is the key for long-term success. In this

Fig 12-12 The influence of professional oral care on caries and periodontitis after 6 years. (Data taken from Axelsson and Lindhe.[14])

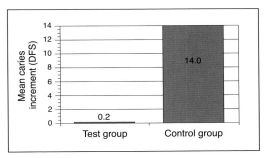

Fig 12-12a New cavities after 6 years. (DFS = decayed or filled surfaces.)

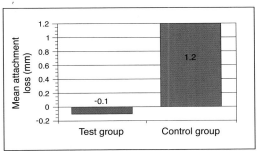

Fig 12-12b Mean attachment loss (all sites) after 6 years. Note that in the test group, there was even a small gain in attachment.

phase, the patient is taken into a well-organized recall system, where, depending on the individual risk, the patient sees a dental hygienist 15 to 65 times per year. During the appointments, both the restorations and the oral hygiene status are evaluated. The patient receives further motivation and instruction in oral hygiene techniques as needed. Then the teeth are professionally cleaned and fluoride is applied. With such a regimen, the dental office is able to maintain oral health over years.

The maintenance phase was shown to be effective in the classic study by Axelsson and Lindhe,[14] in which patients received complete reconstructions in 1972. Afterward, they were split into two groups. The patients in the test group attended a professional recall appointment as described 45 times per year, while the patients in the control group were told to see their clinician for a cleaning once a year. The results of maintenance visits after 6 years were dramatic (Fig 12-12).

The study population was observed for 30 years. In 1978 the control group was eliminated for ethical reasons, and all of those patients were given individual risk-related preventive care. From 1978 until 2002, 60% of the patients in the test group saw the dental hygienist once per year, 30% attended maintenance visits twice per year, and 10% of the patients required only 3 to 4 visits per year. Of the initial 375 patients, 257 were checked after 30 years. The age distribution of the three groups at that time was as follows: group 1, 50 to 65 years old; group 2, 66 to 80 years old; and group 3, 81 to 95 years old. In 1972 the average number of teeth present per individual (all groups) was 25.7. After 30 years the average number of teeth was 25.1, which means that only 0.6 tooth per individual was lost during this time period; in other words, approximately every second patient lost one tooth in 30 years (Axelsson P, personal communication, 2003).

The Solution: Biotechnology

The future of dentistry will not lie in more and more sophisticated technologies for restorations. Certainly, future restorative materials and techniques will yield restorations for the patient's lifetime. However, the factors that are responsible for the diseases will still be latent. Changes in patients' lives may produce recurrence of disease. Therefore, it is better to find ways to inhibit the diseases and to develop methods to reconstruct teeth close to the way nature created them. In 1988 a method was proposed for removing decayed tissue by dissolution and subsequent colonization of the site with modified microorganisms that are able to produce dentin and enamel.[15] With this mechanism it should be possible to create "natural" restorations.

Hillmann et al[16] have modified streptococci mutans such that the endpoint of their metabolic pathway is alcohol instead of lactate. Consequently, plaque that contains mainly this subspecies will not be cariogenic. This could be a lifelong mechanism to prevent caries if the modified streptococci are inoculated into the oral cavity before the unmodified bacteria are prevalent.

Another possibility is to find or develop substances that will modify the pellicle in such a way that microorganisms will not adhere to the tooth. A mouthrinse containing such a substance would at least temporarily protect teeth from being colonized. Understanding the quorum-sensing mechanism of the bacteria in microbial plaques, one could create a mouthrinse that would dissolve plaque.[17]

The better we understand biology, the more specific we can be in our treatments to benefit oral health. Imagine saliva glands that would also produce substances that prevent microorganisms from colonizing on the teeth, such as antibodies against *Streptococcus mutans* or periodontal pathogens. With the advances of molecular biology and gene technology, such solutions are not out of reach.

References

1. Mjör I. Placement and replacement of restorations. Oper Dent 1981;6:49–54.

2. Klausner LH, Green TG, Charbenau GT. Placement and replacement of amalgam restorations. A challenge for the profession. Oper Dent 1987;12:105–112.

3. König KG. Karies und Parodontopathien. Ätiologie und Prophylaxe. Stuttgart: Thieme, 1987.

4. Thylstrup A, Fejerskov O. Textbook of Cariology. Copenhagen: Munksgaard, 1986.

5. Axelsson P, Lindhe J. Effect of oral hygiene instruction and professional toothcleaning on caries and gingivitis in schoolchildren. Community Dent Oral Epidemiol 1981;9:251–255.

6. Weinstein P, Milgrom P, Melnick S, Beach B, Spadafora A. How effective is oral hygiene instruction? Results after 6 and 24 weeks. J Public Health Dent 1989;49:32–38.

7. Zimmer S, Didner B, Roulet J-F. Clinical study on the plaque-removing ability of a new triple-headed toothbrush. J Clin Periodontol 1999;26: 281–285.

8. Zimmer S, Fosca M, Roulet J-F. Clinical study of the effectiveness of two sonic toothbrushes. J Clin Dent 2000;11:24–27.

9. Imfeld TN. Identification of Low Caries Risk Dietary Components. Basel, Switzerland: Karger, 1983.

10. Gustafsson BE, Quensel CE, Swenander Lanke L, et al. The effect of different levels of carbohydrate intake on caries activity in 436 individuals observed for 5 years. Acta Odontol Scand 1954;11:232–364.

11. Haller B, Blunck U. Übersicht und Wertung der aktuellen Bondingsysteme. Zahnarztl Mitt 2003; 93:808–818.

12. Kanzler R, Roulet J-F. Margin quality and longevity in vivo of sintered ceramic inlays luted with adhesive techniques. In: Mörmann WH (ed). CAD/CIM in Aesthetic Dentistry. Chicago: Quintessence, 1996:537–552.

13. Lang NP. Checkliste Zahnärztliche Behandlungsplanung, ed 2. Stuttgart: Auflage Thieme, 1988.

14. Axelsson P, Lindhe J. Effect of controlled oral hygiene procedures on caries and periodontal diseases in adults. J Clin Periodontol 1981;8: 239–248.

15. Roulet J-F. Zukunftsaspekte der Zahnerhaltung. Swiss Dent 1988;9:23–33.

16. Hillmann JD, Brooks TA, Michalek SM, Harmon CC, Snoep JL, van der Weijden CC. Construction and characterization of an effector strain of *Streptococcus mutans* for replacement therapy of dental caries. Infect Immun 2000;13:108–125.

17. Costerton JW, Stewart PS, Greenberg EP. Bacterial biofilms, a common cause of persistent infections. Science 1999;284:1318–1322.

Index